Phantom Voices, Ethereal Music &
other Spooky Sounds

Musical Ear Syndrome

*Unraveling the Mysteries of the Auditory Hallucinations
Many Hard of Hearing People Secretly Experience*

Phantom Voices, Ethereal Music & other Spooky Sounds

Musical Ear Syndrome

Unraveling the Mysteries of the Auditory Hallucinations Many Hard of Hearing People Secretly Experience

Neil G. Bauman, Ph.D.

GuidePost Publications

Stewartstown, PA   http://www.GuidePostPublications.com

Phantom Voices, Ethereal Music & other Spooky Sounds

Musical Ear Syndrome: Unraveling the Mysteries of the Auditory Hallucinations

Many Hard of Hearing People Secretly Experience

Another **GuidePost** book in the series:

Everything You Wanted to Know About Your Hearing Loss But Were Afraid to Ask
(Because You Knew You Wouldn't Hear the Answers Anyway!)

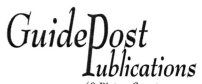

GuidePost Publications

49 Piston Court,
Stewartstown, PA 17363-8322
Phone: (717) 993-8555
FAX: (717) 993-6661
E-mail: info@GuidePostPublications.com
Website: http://www.GuidePostPublications.com

Printed in the United States of America

Warning–Disclaimer

This book is for your education and reference. It is neither a medical manual nor a guide to self-treatment for medical problems. Do not construe this book as giving personal medical advice or instruction. The author is not a medical doctor and neither prescribes treatment nor treats medical problems and does not intend that you attempt to do so either. If you suspect that you have a medical problem related to your ears, seek competent professional medical help. Use the information in this book to help you make informed decisions, not as a substitute for any treatment that your doctor may have prescribed for you.

The information and opinions expressed in this book are the result of careful research. They are believed to be accurate and sound, based on the best judgment available to the author. If you fail to consult appropriate health professionals, you assume the risk of any injuries. Neither GuidePost Publications nor the author assumes any responsibility for damages or losses incurred as a result of using the information in this book, nor for any errors or omissions. It is the responsibility of each reader to exercise good judgment in using any information contained in this book.

Trademarks

Trademarked names appear in this book. Rather than list the names and entities that own the trademarks, or insert a trademark symbol with each mention of the trademarked name, the publisher states that it is using the names with no intention of infringing upon that trademark. To this end, all the brand names of drugs and chemicals are printed in italics with the initial letter capitalized. These brand names are the registered trademarks of their respective pharmaceutical and chemical companies.

About the Author

Neil G. Bauman, Ph.D., (Dr. Neil) is the executive director of the Center for Hearing Loss Help in Pennsylvania. He is a hearing loss coping skills specialist, researcher, author and speaker on issues pertaining to hearing loss. No stranger to hearing loss himself, he has lived with a life-long severe hereditary hearing loss.

Dr. Neil did not let his hearing loss stop him from achieving what he wanted to do. He earned several degrees in fields ranging from forestry to ancient astronomy (Ph.D.) and theology (Th.D.). Later, he trained as a hearing loss coping skills specialist.

For the past number of years, Dr. Neil has researched a variety of hearing loss issues, including the effects of ototoxic drugs on people, and the phantom sounds many hard of hearing people experience.

His mission is helping hard of hearing people understand and successfully cope with their hearing losses. To this end, he provides education, support and counsel to hard of hearing people through personal contact, as well as through his books, presentations and seminars.

Dr. Neil is the author of ten books and a wide variety of articles on hearing-loss related topics. (See the back of this book for a list of his books.) In addition, he is a dynamic speaker. His presentations are in demand throughout the USA and Canada.

You can reach him at:

Neil Bauman
49 Piston Court
Stewartstown, PA   17363
Phone: (717) 993-8555
FAX: (717) 993-6661
Email: neil@hearinglosshelp.com
Website: http://www.hearinglosshelp.com

I dedicate this book to
the many people
who shared their stories
of hearing phantom sounds with me,
so that
this book might help those
who experience
Musical Ear syndrome
to better understand what is often
a scary and anxiety-laden experience.

Contents

Preface

Hallucinations—the very term conjures up visions of phantom voices, padded cells and people in white coats talking in hushed tones. This is because most people associate hallucinations with "going crazy" and mental illness.

In spite of the "bad press" hallucinations have received, the truth is, hearing phantom voices, ethereal music and other spooky sounds does **not** necessarily mean a person is mentally ill. It's time to demystify the subject of auditory hallucinations— to separate myth from fact.

Since I am neither a medical doctor nor a psychiatrist, I do not diagnosis or treat medical/psychotic conditions. Therefore, if you experience auditory hallucinations as a result of a medical disorder, pathological brain condition or mental illness such as schizophrenia, seek competent medical help. This book is **not** meant for you.

On the other hand, if you hear hallucinations, but are otherwise "normal," this book can help you understand the phantom sounds you hear and will show you various ways you can help yourself reduce or eliminate them.

As you read this book, you likely will be surprised to discover that you are not alone. In fact, **thousands** of other people hear the same phantom sounds you do.

If you are a doctor or other health care professional, realize this book is written from the perspective of people who hear auditory hallucinations. It gives rare insight into what they actually experience, and into how they perceive your attitudes towards them when they reveal that they "hear voices." The examples in this book tell it like it is as they see it. Unfortunately, these same examples reveal that many doctors do not have the knowledge and concern they should have regarding auditory hallucinations. It further reveals some major shortcomings health care professionals have in regards to effectively diagnosing and treating auditory hallucinations.

The blame is not all on the shoulders of the medical community, however. Hard of hearing people who experience auditory hallucinations are also part of the problem. This is because hard of hearing people seldom talk to anyone about the phantom sounds they hear for fear of being thought crazy. You, as health care professionals, on the other hand, have failed to take this condition seriously and often believe people experiencing auditory hallucinations really are psychotic. Can you blame them for shutting you out?

My desire is that this book will bring both sides together—that it will bring knowledge and understanding to both the health care professionals and to the many people who suffer from non-psychiatric auditory hallucinations.

All the stories in this book are true. I could never "dream up" such interesting and diverse accounts on my own. In many of these stories, it seems that the truth is stranger than fiction. Nevertheless, that is the way it really is. Each of these stories is in the person's own words, although I have edited these stories for brevity and clarity. All names are real unless I use a pseudonym (name shown in quotes) in order to protect a person's identity. Thus, Sam would be a storyteller's real name, but "Jane" would be a pseudonym.

People around the world have sent me these stories. As a result, the Susan you read about may just as easily live in Australia, or South Africa, or Great Britain, or Canada, or any other country as in the United States. Often several people have the same first names, so the Susan you read about in one story may or may not be the same Susan you encounter in another place.

I thank the many people who have given me permission to tell their stories. Indeed, many were glad to have me tell their stories. These stories will be a tremendous help to people encountering the baffling mysteries of auditory hallucinations for the first time.

Finally, if you are hard of hearing, look on the bright side. Hearing auditory hallucinations isn't all bad. Where else can you hear beautiful music without hearing aids, assistive devices, players, headphones or other paraphernalia?

Neil Bauman, Ph.D.
Stewartstown, PA
January, 2005

Chapter 1

Sane or Psychotic—What Do You Think?

Few people openly dare to mention hearing phantom voices, ethereal music or other spooky noises, yet a surprising number do hear these strange phantom sounds.

Following are ten of their stories. As you read each of these accounts, ask yourself, "Is this person sane or psychotic?" In other words, in your opinion, does this person need help from a psychiatrist or is this just a sane person who happens to be experiencing "weird" hearing?

Case 1: Shirley writes:

Recently, I became deaf. I was awakened in the middle of the night by what I thought were people calling to me. I became truly frightened when I realized that I was deaf and should not be able to hear voices. Now I hear something akin to rap music as well as environmental sounds such as phones ringing or footsteps.

Is Shirley sane or psychotic?

Case 2: "Helen" recounts:

I have a 98% hearing loss in my right ear and about 80% in the left. About a year and a half ago, I started being awakened at night by very loud "2-way radio" voices in my right ear. These radio voices generally occur when I'm asleep and are so loud in my deaf ear they wake me up. Sometimes I even jump. It happens every night.

It is rather scary because we live in the country, and I thought maybe it was drug dealers with sophisticated communication equipment. Every night I now hear our county deputy on his radio. It's annoying and scary because I can distinguish enough of the conversations to hear phrases such as "armed with a knife" and "body of male discovered." This morning the deputy was singing a little rap song when he received a call. Sometimes I also hear music which I believe is the road crew passing the house in the early morning hours. In no way is this an hallucination.

Is "Helen" sane or psychotic?

Case 3: Years ago, when she was a girl, "Sherry" recalled:

When my dad would take me flying in his little two-seater wind-knocker airplane, I used to hear strange music. The music sounded like the full Mormon Tabernacle Choir. Since I was very young, I thought it was angels singing.

Was "Sherry" sane or psychotic?

Case 4: Carolyn, a senior, explains:

Late at night when I don't have my hearing aids on, I am sure I hear motors of large trucks working right outside our bedroom windows. We are the only ones living on our little country lane. There's no traffic of any kind outside my bedroom windows. My husband swears there are no noises at all.

Is Carolyn sane or psychotic?

Case 5: Nancy relates:

My neighbor is 71 and has lost most of her hearing. She lives alone and hears phantom music often. The problem is, she hears motorcycles outside her home at different times but usually every night. She says she also hears men talking and fighting outside her home. They beat on her window and the walls of her house at times. She said they had gotten on top of her house two nights ago.

She calls the police and myself and another neighbor that tries to look after her, and we can never find anything that would indicate anyone was there. We live in a good neighborhood that has never had these type of problems. We have even spent the night at her home and heard nothing.

Is Nancy's neighbor sane or psychotic?

Case 6: Jane is 49 and has normal hearing. She explains:

For years I've been "hearing" music of various sorts when I lay in bed waiting to go to sleep—from band and orchestral, to Irish folk music, symphony and opera. Now I hear phantom music almost all the time—at home, while I'm driving, at work—except when I am actively engaged at a task. I hear passages of what sounds like Strauss waltzes, Russian symphonies and Italian operas distinctively enough to identify various instruments, male or female choruses, and the occasional soloist.

Is Jane sane or psychotic?

Case 7: Rose is 80 years old and writes:

I hear radio weather reports! My house overlooks a harbor where boats and ships sometimes anchor. I only hear this when a vessel is anchored—not when the harbor is empty. Although I am profoundly deaf, even without my aids I can clearly hear a man's voice saying "Good morning, good morning. This is WNEW and then words about cloudy, windy and temperature, etc., but not as clearly." The "report" is repeated over and over and over again! This afternoon, I also briefly heard a woman's voice (no good morning) with the call letters WINS. Both WNEW and WINS are actual radio call letters here. This has been going on for several days.

Is Rose sane or is she now psychotic?

Case 8: "Zelda," a student, relates:

Lately I've been hearing voices. I don't know where they come from but they are loud and clear. Last week, for example, I was sitting in class when this voice told me that the boy sitting behind me was planning to attack me after school. I jumped out of my seat and began to scream obscenities at him. He denied everything, of course, so I hit him and broke his nose.[1]

Is "Zelda" sane or psychotic?

Case 9: Marcy writes:

I had just come back in from going outside to tell my husband that I was really afraid I was becoming schizoid. The first phantom song I heard was *America the Beautiful*, followed by *Amazing Grace*. Since then, I've heard phantom songs almost constantly while awake for the last 7 days, with about 6 different general tunes. This music has been getting a bit louder with time. In fact, if I cover my ears, I can still "hear" it, and my talking doesn't quite alleviate it either. This morning for instance, I've heard the hymn *How Great Thou Art*—or at least repetitive portions of some such—all morning long.

Is Marcy sane or psychotic?

Case 10: "Dennis" states:

I heard voices almost nonstop for 2 years. At first, it was just two voices inside my head talking to each other. Later, more voices joined in the conversations, some of them from outside my head. I thought I could talk to the voices with my mind, but no one heard me talking

[1] Ask the Expert—Auditory Hallucinations, 1999. p. 1.

19

to them. Some of the voices started telling me what to do. At first, they tried to make me do benign things, like play on the computer. Then they became nastier. They insisted that I hurt or kill myself or other people. They taunted me in class and talked about me to each other like I wasn't even there.[2]

Is "Dennis" sane or psychotic?

How did you do? If you decided that the people in cases 1-7 and 9 are sane, although each hears strange phantom sounds that supposedly normal people do not hear, you are correct. In addition, if you believe that the people in cases 8 and 10 have problems with mental illness, you are also correct.

[2] Long, 2003. p. 3.

Chapter 2

Distinguishing Psychiatric from Non-Psychiatric Auditory Hallucinations

Exactly what are hallucinations? Hallucinations are "the apparent, often strong, subjective perception of an object or event when no such stimulus or situation is present."[1] Put another way, hallucinations are (phantom) sensory phenomena in the absence of (real) external sensory stimuli.[2]

Thus, hallucinations are where your brain perceives something is happening even though your five senses have not received any external stimulus. Hallucinations may be visual (seeing), auditory (hearing), olfactory (smelling), gustatory (tasting) or tactile (feeling). Therefore, hallucinations are simply seeing, hearing, smelling, tasting or feeling sights, sounds, odors, tastes, or sensations that no one else around you perceives.

Although hallucinations may occur with any of the five senses, auditory hallucinations are by far the most common kind of hallucination.[4] A person is hearing auditory hallucinations when he or she hear noises, music, sounds or voices that no one else hears. Auditory hallucinations can be pleasant, neutral or frightening.[5]

People who experience auditory hallucinations may be sane (and many are), or they may be psychotic (have a mental illness). This is because there are two basic kinds of auditory hallucinations—psychiatric auditory hallucinations and non-psychiatric auditory hallucinations.

Hallucinations

The term hallucination is from the Latin *alucinari* which means "to wander in the mind." It was first introduced into psychiatric literature back in 1837.[3]

[1] Stedman's Medical Dictionary, 2000. p. 784.

[2] Roberts, 2001. p. 423.

[3] Boza, 1999. p. 2.

[4] Eizenberg, 1987. p. 3.

[5] Hallucinations, 2002. p. 2.

Psychiatric auditory hallucinations are hallucinations arising from a mental illness and are so named because psychiatrists typically treat these conditions. Some doctors refer to them as **pathologic** hallucinations since mental illness, to their minds, is a pathologic condition of the mind.

In contrast, non-psychiatric auditory hallucinations have nothing whatsoever to do with mental illness. These hallucinations include **psychological** events, **physiological** conditions and **pharmacological** reactions.

Psychological events are sometimes called **psychological** hallucinations or **non-pathological** hallucinations.[6] These are the kinds of hallucinations many hard of hearing people experience from time to time. Physiological conditions (technically also pathological hallucinations) include hallucinations arising from physical problems in the brain such as brain tumors. Pharmacological reactions include auditory hallucinations caused by various "recreational," prescription and over-the-counter drugs.

In summary, auditory hallucinations result from one of these four primary causes, namely:
1. mental illness,
2. abnormal brain conditions/diseases
3. drug side effects, or
4. something not working quite right in the auditory system.

Thus, it is wrong to lump all auditory hallucinations together under a psychiatric label. It is just as wrong to lump them all together under the non-psychiatric label. These are two distinct conditions. Of course, auditory hallucinations may result from a combination of any, or all, of the above.

In this book, I refer to auditory hallucinations that are connected with mental illness as **psychiatric auditory hallucinations**. I lump the other auditory hallucinations that have nothing to do with mental illness (including psychological, physiological and pharmacological auditory hallucinations) under the banner of **non-psychiatric auditory hallucinations**. This avoids confusion, since, to the average person, the terms "psychiatric" and "psychological" are somewhat synonymous.

[6] Hoffman, 2003. pp. 1-2.

Psychiatric Auditory Hallucinations

Psychiatric auditory hallucinations are signs of mental illness—what psychiatrists like to call a psychosis. The most common kind of mental illness associated with hearing psychiatric auditory hallucinations is schizophrenia. About 70% of the people with schizophrenia and about 15% of the people with mood disorders such as mania or depression hear such hallucinations.[7]

The auditory hallucinations associated with schizophrenia are almost exclusively those of speech (voices) rather than music or other sounds.[9]

One type of auditory hallucination peculiar to people with schizophrenia is where the person hears his own thoughts out loud and feels that everyone can hear him thinking his most private thoughts.[10]

Sometimes the person may recognize the voice they are hearing as that of a family member, a deceased friend, a stranger or even God. The voices may be those of dead, fictional, historical or living people.[11] Of the 56% that recognized the voices they heard, 30% were of friends, 29% were of family, 14% were religious (angels, God), and 13% were occult.

Though these voices arise internally, the person "hearing" them feels he is hearing the voice of another.[12] 51% said they heard the voices inside their heads, 40% said outside, and 9% said it was a combination of the two. The voices may also seem to originate from inanimate objects—the walls, the ground, a tree, a shoe, etc.[13]

People with schizophrenia commonly hear a voice or voices speaking to, or about, them. Of the patients who reported hearing conversations, 36% described the conversations as being about them while 29% described the conversations as including them, in that they spoke to their voices, and their voices spoke back to them. In a study of 87 people with known mental illness, 7% heard commands, 48% overheard conversations regarding themselves, and 61% noted being called names.

Psychosis

A psychosis is "a mental and behavioral disorder causing gross distortion or disorganization of a person's mental capacity, affective response, and capacity to recognize reality, communicate, and relate to others to the degree of interfering with the person's capacity to cope with the ordinary demands of everyday life."[8]

Psychotic

Psychotic means: relating to or affected by a psychosis.

[7] Hoffman, 2003. p. 1.

[8] Stedman's Medical Dictionary, 2000. p. 1478.

[9] McKay, 2002. p. 1.

[10] Fadirepo, ~2002. pp. 3-4.

[11] Hallucinations, 2002. p. 2.

[12] Cohen, 1995. p. 1.

[13] Fadirepo, ~2002. p. 3.

These phantom voices often refer to them in the third person calling them worthless, useless or no-good. Sometimes there is a running commentary, while at other times they hear whispers. For example, 19% heard a narrative of their actions, 34% heard accusations, 34% heard threats, while 31% reported hearing niceties.[14]

The voices are often vulgar or derogatory ("You are a fat whore!" "Go to hell!") In the worst cases, the voices command the person to commit suicide or kill someone.[15]

Here are three examples of psychiatric auditory hallucinations. "Daisy" said:

> I started hearing three male voices commenting on my behavior and sometimes judging me, calling me useless and lazy. Now I just hear one voice telling me over and over again to cut myself and kill myself.[16]

"Linda" relates:

> Recently I have been hearing a specific voice, a very evil deep man's voice. It started out sounding like the devil's voice, then it started talking to me, most of the time very degrading negative comments. When I was in my car driving home, I was so terrified of it and I was so scared, I just kept driving. The voice then told me to kill myself in a slow, painful way.[17]

"Kristy" explains:

> My voices taunt me and ridicule me and eventually I want to kill myself because they convince me that is the only thing I can do. In addition, I have also had the voices telling me that I have to kill my son because I shouldn't hurt him by leaving him here on earth.[18]

As you will soon discover, these experiences differ vastly from the experiences of many hard of hearing people who hear the non-psychiatric kind of auditory hallucinations.

How can a person tell apart an inspired voice (God or an angel), an isolated instance of hearing one's own name being called (possibly an anxiety reflex), and the voices mentally ill people hear? One answer is that clearly-understandable non-pathological (non-psychiatric) voices occur rarely or perhaps only once. Not so for a mentally ill person. Without treatment, their voices recur relentlessly.[19]

[14] Holland, ~2001. p.2.

[15] Hoffman, 2003. p. 1.

[16] Long, 2003. p. 1.

[17] Long, 2003. p. 2.

[18] Long, 2003. p. 2.

[19] Hoffman, 2003. pp. 1-2.

Incidentally, people who experience various non-psychiatric hallucinations soon learn from experience that their hallucinations are not real. On the other hand, mentally-ill people generally have difficulty separating their hallucinations from reality.[20]

This is all I am going to say about psychiatric auditory hallucinations. The remainder of this book deals exclusively with non-psychiatric auditory hallucinations.

Note: In order to simplify things, from now on I will generally refer to non-psychiatric auditory hallucinations as simply auditory hallucinations. Any further references to psychiatric auditory hallucinations will be explicitly stated as such.

Non-Psychiatric Auditory Hallucinations

Non-psychiatric auditory hallucinations, as their name implies, have nothing whatsoever to do with mental illness. There are a few published reports of elderly people who both hear auditory hallucinations (commonly referred to as musical hallucinations), and have a hearing loss. The hallmark of this group is the complete lack of **psychopathology**.[21] In other words, these people are **not** mentally ill.

Lenore's father-in-law fits this profile exactly. After extensive testing, both his physical condition and his mental status checked out just fine. This is in spite of the fact that he hears phantom sounds and appears to act irrationally. She writes:

> My father-in-law has been hard of hearing for some time. He hears auditory hallucinations. **His MRI, EEG and CT scan were all normal. The geriatric psychiatrist tested him and found no dementia.** He mainly hears loud music when **alone** in his apartment, oftentimes in the middle of the night. Unfortunately, he has taken to knocking on the downstairs landlady's door (at 3 A.M.) telling her to turn the music down. We have been with him a few times when he heard the music—none of us heard anything.

Auditory hallucinations associated with hearing loss are **rarely** described in the medical literature. Furthermore, an association between hearing loss and mental disorders in old age has generally **been assumed** but has been **poorly substantiated** in the psychiatric literature.[22] This is a back-handed way of saying that the people who experience auditory

[20] Charles Bonnet Syndrome, 2004. p. 3.

[21] Eizenberg, 1987. p. 3.

[22] Eizenberg, 1987. p. 1.

hallucinations are perfectly sane even though many doctors, because of their ignorance concerning auditory hallucinations, think otherwise.

It is patently ridiculous to assume that people are demented just because they hear auditory hallucinations.[23] So often you read things like, "Auditory hallucinations, with the exception of religious experiences, are abnormal and usually occur in schizophrenia,"[24] as though there was no other alternative.

Quite often, in published reports, the authors try to distinguish between what they call auditory hallucinations (meaning psychiatric auditory hallucinations) and musical hallucinations (meaning non-psychiatric auditory hallucinations). They fail to realize that although the majority of non-psychiatric auditory hallucinations have some musical qualities, they also include hearing voices and other sounds of a non-psychiatric kind. One writer points out:

> These hallucinations are **not** the same as those associated with those of psychotic individuals in which they hear voices with **meaningful content**.[25]

A key to understanding one basic difference between psychiatric and non-psychiatric auditory hallucinations is in the words "meaningful content." People with psychiatric auditory hallucinations hear voices speaking **to or about them**. In contrast, when people experience non-psychiatric auditory hallucinations, any voices they hear are often vague and the content is of a **general**, not personal, nature. They may hear what sounds vaguely like a radio broadcast. For example, Malisa explained:

> I get Red Barber calling the game, I can't distinguish the words—but I'm sure that's who is talking.

Dora had a similar experience. She related:

> I heard what sounded like the voice of a radio announcer on a badly tuned radio station.

These are often the kinds of voices people with non-psychiatric auditory hallucinations typically "hear."

[23] Edell, 1998. p. 1.

[24] Hallucinations, 2002. p. 2.

[25] Tinnitus, ~2004. p. 6.

Chapter 3

Some Characteristics of Auditory Hallucinations

Auditory hallucinations cover an enormous range of sound experiences. They may consist of simple or complex sounds. These sounds may be formed or unformed. Sometimes the person hearing auditory hallucinations knows he is hearing phantom sounds. Even stranger, sometimes auditory hallucinations may piggyback themselves on real sounds.

Simple vs. Complex Sounds (Tinnitus vs. Auditory Hallucinations)

Auditory hallucinations can be broken down into two groups of sounds based on their complexity. **Simple** sounds are basically single, unmodulated sounds such as the various tinnitus sounds millions of people hear (see sidebar). In fact, tinnitus is the most common kind of auditory hallucination people hear.

Tinnitus sounds may be subjective or objective. Subjective tinnitus sounds are only "heard" by the person experiencing them. As such, they are a form of auditory hallucinations. Objective tinnitus sounds (such as those related to the heart beat or clicking sounds from the middle ear) can be heard by other people. These sounds are not hallucinatory, but are real sounds. However, the vast majority of people with tinnitus experience the subjective variety.

Tinnitus sounds

Tinnitus manifests itself as a wide variety of simple sounds. Tinnitus may sound like ringing, roaring, beating, clicking, banging, buzzing, hissing, humming, blowing, chirping, clanging, sizzling, whooshing, rumbling, whistling or dreadful shrieking noises in your head. Tinnitus may also sound like rushing water, radio static, breaking glass, bells ringing, owls hooting or chainsaws running.[1]

[1] Bauman, 2002. p. 7.

The thing that distinguishes subjective tinnitus from other phantom sounds is that although tinnitus may have a tonal quality, it is always a simple sound—basically a monotone.

In contrast to the simple sounds of tinnitus, **complex** sounds include multiple, modulated sounds such as tunes, singing, music and voices.[2] These are the sounds that are traditionally called auditory hallucinations.

Auditory hallucinations arise from a different place in our brains than tinnitus. However, their effect may be much the same. That is why many people think the musical sounds they hear are just another form of tinnitus. Linda thought this. She wrote:

> **I had always considered the snatches of song and voices (unintelligible) to be just another form of tinnitus**. This stuff is all my head plays. I rarely get other phantom noises. It's always music and voices.

"Valerie" wondered whether the more complex musical and vocal sounds she heard was a strange kind of tinnitus. She questioned:

> I have tinnitus all the time. Sometimes I even hear what sounds like music or people singing or talking. **Is this some strange kind of tinnitus**?

Phyllis wondered much the same thing. She asked:

> I know that I have auditory hallucinations. My question is: **Is it still considered tinnitus?**

The truth is, tinnitus is a type of auditory hallucination—not the other way around. What these ladies are hearing is the complex sounds of auditory hallucinations in addition to their usual tinnitus.

Unformed vs. Formed Auditory Hallucinations

Depending on how "clear" they are, phantom sounds are referred to as being either "unformed" or "formed."

Unformed auditory hallucinations consist of hearing distorted (complex) noises, music, sounds, or voices.[3] These sounds are vague, "fuzzy" and indistinct. Notice the vague

[2] Wade, 1995. p. 26.

[3] Hallucinations, 2002. p. 2.

quality in the descriptions of the following examples of unformed auditory hallucinations.

Robin described her unformed auditory hallucinations as:

...like the wind blowing, but with a musical quality, as if someone off in the distance was singing without words.

"Elizabeth" said:

I've never heard a tune that I could identify. It sounds more like an orchestra warming up.

Carolina described hers thus:

When I am in a real quiet room I hear this humming in my head like someone is humming a song but can't keep a tune.

Steve described his as:

...some song that sounds for all the world like it belongs as a theme song for PBS, but I can't place it.

Karen relates:

I sometimes hear phantom "radio broadcasts" that I can't quite make out.

Chris explains:

The words are never distinct—it's like they are several rooms away.

Sometimes the music may be familiar, although the words may be indistinguishable. For example, one person, who had been hard of hearing for 5 years, heard auditory hallucinations:

...in the form of multiple singers singing familiar melodies with indistinguishable voices. The songs included hymns, rugby songs and recent popular music.[4]

Another lady had been hearing unformed auditory hallucinations for 10 years. She experienced musical hallucinations in which:

...the individual notes had the quality of a buzzy pitch. Her experience had evolved from almost continuous tinnitus with similar characteristics to the buzzy pitches experienced as music.[5]

Diana also hears vague and less clearly-formed auditory hallucinations. She explains:

Some evenings I am "treated" to a few hours of continuous classical music from various periods and styles. I have searched this house

[4] Griffiths, 2000. p. 2066.
[5] Griffiths, 2000. p. 2067.

over. I looked for a radio left plugged in somewhere. It sounds exactly like music or TV in another room that's just enough outside of hearing range that you can't pin it down.

Tonight I heard a long Wagnerian sort of opera piece, and later, a lot of rolling trills on the piano, ala Gershwin. Sometimes I get County, Pop or Gospel flavors too, but **all I can sense are the flavors, not fully identifiable**. I can distinguish the trumpet fanfares from the violin movements from the orchestral drum passages. When it's voices, I may hear repetitive chanting, or DJ-like banter, or news/weather drone, etc. Once in a great while I do get an identifiable clear word or two, usually in a voice I don't recall ever hearing. Last night it was a very lyrical woman's voice and she said something like "tho mani tho" whatever that is.

In contrast, **formed** auditory hallucinations are where speech or music is clear and recognizable. For example, Don hears clearly-formed auditory hallucinations. He recounts his experiences:

For the past 3 to 4 months I have had the most calming and repetitive choruses and wind ensembles, usually led by a bass sax and a baritone, playing and singing in a low octave, the older Christian hymns and a few oldies from the forties such as, *Near the Cross*, *Amazing Grace*, *His Eye Is on the Sparrow* and *The Star Spangled Banner*.

Jane also hears clearly-formed auditory hallucinations. She writes:

I hear passages of what sound like Strauss waltzes, Russian symphonies, Italian operas—distinctively enough to identify various instruments, male or female choruses, and the occasional soloist.

One person, who had been hard of hearing for 40 years, heard auditory hallucinations consisting of light operatic pieces and popular songs by artists including British singer Shirley Bassey and Boyzone.[6]

Another person, also with a hearing loss for the past 40 years, heard organ or piano music, sometimes accompanied by singers. If accompanied by singers, the lyrics would be distinguishable. The songs included hymns, nursery rhymes and old popular songs.[7]

Interestingly enough, some people's auditory hallucinations seem to swing back and forth, sometimes being clearly formed and other times becoming vague and unformed. Here is how Carol describes hers.

[6] Griffiths, 2000. pp. 2066-7.
[7] Griffiths, 2000. p. 2067.

What I hear is music only, no voices, and it is very definitely a brass band with the trombones dominating, although I hear cornets off and on. The music is identifiable about 80% - 90% of the time. What I hear most is *The Battle Hymn of the Republic*, *Auld Lang Syne*, *In Your Easter Bonnet*, *Rock of Ages*, *Abide With Me*, and occasionally *It's a Grand Old Flag*. When a piece fades out there is often applause and cheering (muted, to be sure) and then it starts all over again. They aren't necessarily complete pieces, but repetitions of key themes or refrains. Of the pieces I can't identify, they sound vaguely familiar. For the most part, the songs I hear definitely fall in the clear rather than vague category.

For many people, their auditory hallucinations start off with clearly-formed complete sentences or songs. Later, the repetition of lengthy passages of music may eventually degenerate into short snatches of repetitive phrases or rhythmic patterns. This is what Loretta's mom heard. She writes:

My mother is 92 and has a severe hearing loss in both ears. Recently she began having auditory hallucinations of music at first and **now it is just repetitive nonsense words or phrases**.

David's father's auditory hallucinations also quickly degenerated from the beautiful music it started out as. He explains:

My dad's musical hallucinations started out as recognizable songs (*Battle Hymn of the Republic* for 2 weeks, then started changing to a variety of other songs, *The Music Man*, *Ride of the Valkyries*, etc.) then **turned into unrecognizable orchestral or vocal like (no words) sounds**.

"Mindy" had a somewhat similar experience. She writes:

I hear vague music but it is the same few songs over and over again. They are *Brahms Lullaby*, *America* and *The Happy Wanderer*. If I put my fingers in my ears, I still hear it.

Usually the entire songs play softly, but quite clearly (just the music, not the words). One song plays over and over for a long time, then sometimes it just changes to another, or a few notes change, but its always the same few songs.

A few days later she reported:

Most of last night and this morning, instead of music, I've been hearing the sounds of chords, with the notes of the chords played one at a time up and down, and up and down (like C, up to E, up to G, up to C, down to G, down to E, down to C, up to E, up to G...). Occasionally it will change to another key but keep doing the same exercise as if someone is practicing chords on the piano. Once in a while the chords would stop and *Brahms' Lullaby* would play, but then the chords would start again (which is very monotonous—I think I'd prefer having the old songs back).

A little while ago, the music started again, but this time it was a new song, the *Tennessee Waltz*. Now, after several hours of the *Tennessee Waltz*, with *Brahms' Lullaby* interspersed here and there, the chords are back again. I'm wondering if the little musician in my head is practicing to play another new song.

Often the music initially sounds pleasant, and then over days or weeks, the music degrades in quality so that it sounds like a scratched phonograph record.[8] Marcy explains:

The first phantom song I heard was *America the Beautiful*, followed by *Amazing Grace*. Since then, I've had it almost constantly while awake for the last 7 days, with about 6 different general tunes. This morning, for instance, I've heard the hymn *How Great Thou Art*—or at least **repetitive portions** of some such all morning long.

Roger's auditory hallucinations also degenerated. He wrote:

I began hearing the national anthem being played. Then all of a sudden it went to *Amazing Grace*. Now it is a **repetitive three or four notes**.

Pseudo-Auditory Hallucinations

True auditory hallucinations are phantom sounds you **believe** to be real, but are **not**. In contrast, pseudo or false auditory hallucinations are phantom sounds you **know** to be phantom, even though they **seem** real to you. Therefore, the primary characteristic differentiating true auditory hallucinations from pseudo-auditory hallucinations is whether you are aware of the unreality of your auditory hallucinations.[9]

When people first begin hearing phantom sounds, they think they are real. In truth, they have no reason to believe otherwise because they perceive their phantom sounds as vivid and crisp. Thus, at this point, they are experiencing true auditory hallucinations.

Remember, in Case 2, "Helen" telling of hearing the deputy sheriff on the radio during the night? She explained:

Every night I now hear our county deputy on his radio. It's annoying and scary because I can distinguish enough of the conversations to

Imagined Sounds

Don't confuse auditory hallucinations with imagined sounds. In order to be an auditory hallucination, the sound must appear to be real to you. Thus an imagined sound is not an auditory hallucination since you know that you are not actually hearing it the same way as you normally hear sounds.[10]

[8] Deutsch, 2002. p. 1.

[9] Boza, 1999. p. 7.

[10] Fadirepo, ~2002. p. 3.

hear phrases such as "armed with a knife" and "body of male discovered." This morning the deputy was singing a little rap song when he received a call. In no way is this an hallucination.

Notice her final comment—"**In no way is this an hallucination**." She was totally convinced she was hearing real sounds—so at that point, she was experiencing true auditory hallucinations.

Many other people are just as fooled by their auditory hallucinations. Rick once woke up hearing what sounded like a radio and asked his wife to "turn the darn radio off."

When she first started experiencing auditory hallucinations, Chris couldn't tell her auditory hallucinations apart from reality either. She explains:

I have auditory hallucinations **so real** that on at least two occasions, I have jumped out of bed to investigate things that weren't there!

Often, as time goes on, people begin to realize these sounds are all in their heads—that these are phantom sounds with no external foundation. It is at this point when they realize they are hearing phantom sounds that their auditory hallucinations become pseudo-auditory hallucinations. For example, Margaret writes about her friend Verna:

She has been hearing the music for just one week. At first she heard the music in the bathroom and thought it was coming from the room next door but when she started hearing it in every room she **became aware that it was inside her head**.

Carol came to a similar conclusion. She explains:

For the past few years I have experienced unbidden music on a sporadic basis. Gradually I realized I heard this music at ungodly hours of the night with utter silence outside my window, and that this was **my** problem.

When Karen heard a typewriter clicking away, she would go and check it out to learn whether the sounds were real or phantom. She relates:

I hear a typewriter clicking. It is pretty obnoxious at times. But I hear click.....click, click.......click. Sometimes its fast. Other times its painfully slow. The clicking started when I was about 9 years old. I always thought I was just hearing my mom typing away at the old typewriter she had. I'd go to ask her something and she'd be taking a nap or something.

James came up with a solution to determine whether he was hearing auditory hallucinations or not. He explains:

> I occasionally hear the doorbell ring when I'm lying quietly in bed without my hearing aids on. I thought I was going crazy until a friend told me what was happening. Since then, **I have learned to tell them apart**. If the sound is loud and crystal clear, I answer it. If it's dull and off key, I ignore it. You guys wouldn't believe the number of times I got dressed to answer a phantom doorbell before I figured this out.

Tami, who is 33 and has a hearing loss, writes:

> A few months ago, I began hearing music and "chatter"—unrecognizable and unintelligible muffled murmurings. Almost every time, I know immediately that what I'm hearing isn't real, but I have gone to turn down the radio only to find it wasn't on. Several times I've deferred judgment to my dogs, whose failure to respond to the music/voices told me that it wasn't really there.

Thus in a very real sense, the auditory hallucinations many hard of hearing people experience are really pseudo-auditory hallucinations because they have learned through experience that these sounds are phantom, not real.

However, for the sake of simplicity, I'll generally lump auditory and pseudo-auditory hallucinations together under the term auditory hallucinations since the phantom sounds are the same—it's just the person's awareness of their reality that's different.

Hallucinations Are Not the Same as Illusions

Hallucinations and illusions are not the same. By definition, an illusion is "a false perception; the mistaking of something for what it is not."[12] Illusions are distortions, misperceptions or false impressions of real objects. Thus, illusions are **real** perceptions that are **misinterpreted**. In contrast, hallucinations are where there is **no** real stimulus to mistake for anything else.

If you are unsure whether you are hearing an auditory hallucination or an illusion, ask yourself, "Is this a phantom sound I am hearing, or is it a real sound that I am misinterpreting?" If it is a phantom sound, it is an hallucination. If it is a real sound, then it is an illusion.

Dreams

Both dreams and hallucinations occur when there is decreased external sensory stimuli. They are similar to the extent that a person thinks that the things they are experiencing in their dreams or hallucinations are actually happening.[11] The big difference is that dreams only occur when a person is asleep, while hallucinations require a person to be awake.

[11] Fadirepo, ~2002. p. 15.

[12] Stedman's Medical Dictionary, 2000. p. 876.

A common illusion would be when a ventriloquist and his "dummy" are interacting. The ventriloquist does the actual speaking, but the sound seems to come from the "dummy," not the ventriloquist. Thus you are misinterpreting the source of the sound. You know you are hearing/seeing an illusion.

Here's another example. When I fly, often the steady roar of jet engines eventually turns into a type of music to my ears. There is a real sound (the noise of the jet engines), but I perceive (and my brain eventually misinterprets) it as something else (music). Thus, the music I am hearing is really an illusion. In my case I know what is happening so I am not fooled. However, sometimes the illusion is so good, you don't have a clue you are being fooled. Christine explains:

> My mom, Mary, is hard of hearing. Recently on a trip to Arizona with my dad she commented to dad when they arrived at their hotel that she really enjoyed the music on the plane. Dad said there was no music on the plane. On the return trip, mom started hearing the music again and asked dad, "Don't you hear that music?" He said, "What music?" Mom told him to put on his hearing aids. He did. "Nope, still no music." But mom continued to enjoy it until the plane landed.

In this case, the illusion was so good that Mary didn't have a clue her brain was fooling her into perceiving the jet engine sounds as enjoyable music, thus making the illusion complete.

Chapter 4

How Our Brains Create Auditory Hallucinations

The Brain's Reaction to Sensory Deprivation

God designed our brains with five sensory inputs in order to connect us with our physical environment. Without our five senses, we would be totally isolated from everyone and everything since we would not be able to see, hear, feel, taste or smell people, things or the environment around us.

Because receiving constant sensory input is vital to us, God programmed our brains to constantly monitor sensory inputs. If a sensory organ fails to send a continuous stream of information to our brains, our brains may become "disturbed." When this happens, sometimes, our brains dig deep into their sensory archives and dredge out old memories of these missing senses and somehow use them as inputs in place of the absent sensory inputs.

Thus, if hearing loss causes a lack of sound inputs, our brains may manufacture their own sound tracks. We call these phantom sounds auditory hallucinations. In like manner, if there is a lack of feeling, our brains may manufacture pain and other sensations. If there is a lack of vision, the brains may produce their own "movies."

Following are examples of these phantom sensations. Notice the parallels between them and auditory hallucinations. This will help you better understand the true nature of non-psychiatric auditory hallucinations.

Lack of Feeling—Phantom Limb Syndrome (PLS)

When an accident rips off a person's arm or leg, obviously the sensory inputs going to the brain from that missing limb stop immediately. However, the brain region devoted to that missing limb is still active and can produce a subjective sense of the limb.[1] Thus, even though a person is fully aware of their missing limb, it may still feel like that part of the body is still there—moving, pained, or with other unusual sensations.[2] This is known as Phantom Limb syndrome.

Phantom limb sensations can seem so "real" and lifelike to an amputee that:

> some may attempt to step on a phantom leg and try to walk. When a person with a phantom leg stands up, the phantom leg seems to hang down. It unfolds and stretches out when its owner reclines. It bends properly when its owner sits. When walking, the phantom arm swings in perfect coordination. If a person had a tight ring on a finger or a painful bunion on the foot prior to the amputation of the arm or leg, the tightness is still felt after the amputation.[3]

About 70% of amputees continue to feel sensations of the amputated part. These sensations can include pain, pressure, warmth, cold, itchiness and sweatiness.[4] For example, one man related,

> My grandfather had lost an index finger, but claimed that the end of the missing finger still itched sometimes.

Because such feelings are phantom in that the body part is no longer there, think of Phantom Limb syndrome as a tactile hallucination caused by lack of normal sensory input.[5] In fact, Phantom Limb syndrome was originally called "hallucinated limb."[6] However, today, they have changed the name to Phantom Limb syndrome because these people are not psychotic, even though they experience phantom sensations or hallucinations.

Lack of Seeing—Charles Bonnet Syndrome (CBS)

Perhaps even stranger than Phantom Limb syndrome, is what happens to numerous people when they lose much of their ability to see because of age and/or eye diseases such as

[1] Edell, 1998. p. 1.
[2] Boza, 1999. p. 2.
[3] Juan, 2002. p. 1.
[4] Juan, 2002. p. 1.
[5] Boza, 1999. p. 2.
[6] Juan, 2002. p. 1.

macular degeneration. These people see things that aren't there. Their visual hallucinations take all kinds of forms from simple patterns of straight lines to detailed and vivid pictures of people, buildings[7] and scenery. For example, Steve writes:

> My mother had lost part of her sight (on the right side) to a stroke, but claims to "see" buildings along the side of the road whizzing by when she is riding in a car, even though she knows they are not there.

People who see things that are not there are experiencing visual hallucinations. Again, because of the bad connotation of the word hallucinations, this phenomena goes by the name of Charles Bonnet syndrome (CBS)—named after the man who first described this condition way back in 1760.

Lack of Hearing—Auditory Hallucinations

Since the brain reacts to lack of tactile and visual inputs, it should be no surprise that our brains also react to lack of auditory input. Thus, non-psychiatric auditory hallucinations are to the ears what Charles Bonnet syndrome is to eyes and what Phantom Limb syndrome is to missing arms or legs. Several researchers have seen this parallel. For example:

> Musical hallucinations and Charles Bonnet Syndrome (CBS) have some intriguing similarities to phantom limb syndrome, which involves regional sensory deprivation after the removal of sensory stimuli due to the loss of a limb.[8]

> Musical hallucinations are most commonly seen in subjects with moderate or severe acquired deafness, and as such may **represent an auditory form** of Charles Bonnet syndrome.[9]

> In Charles Bonnet syndrome, because of the absence of normal afferent input [signals from the eyes to the brain], the visual cortex exhibits spontaneous activity, giving rise to conscious imagery. A similar syndrome is found with patients suffering acquired deafness, resulting in musical auditory hallucinations.[10]

> Tinnitus [a type of auditory hallucination] might also be viewed as the auditory-system equivalent to phantom limb pain.[11]

Unfortunately, few people today know about either non-psychiatric auditory hallucinations or Charles Bonnet syndrome. Even fewer see any connection between the two. With rare insight, Kathi asks:

[7] Charles Bonnet Syndrome, 2004. p. 1.

[8] Thorpe, 1997. p 20s.

[9] Griffiths, 2000. p. 2065.

[10] Rahman, 2004. p. 3

[11] Lockwood, 2001. p. 2.

My 83 year old mother has been severely hard of hearing for the past 10 years. She lost her hearing over a period of two years. She has been experiencing auditory hallucinations for several years. My question to you is, have you ever seen visual hallucinations in the same manner? Just recently, within the past month, she has been describing such hallucinations coming from the side view of her right eye. They sound very similar to the auditory hallucinations she has had. The come more often when she is tired, later in the day or evening and when she is alone, which is often.

Although it may not be common, some hard of hearing people with visual problems do experience both Charles Bonnet syndrome and non-psychiatric auditory hallucinations at the same time.[12] Thus, they both see and hear phantom things.

Appendix 1 reveals 22 amazing parallels between non-psychiatric auditory hallucinations and Charles Bonnet syndrome.

A Technical Explanation of Auditory Hallucinations

Research continues into exactly how our brains process sound. Processing sound signals is not a simple process. In fact, just the cortical representation of hearing is highly complex, containing considerable parallel processing, and involves at least 4 cortical levels including 15 or more areas in the brain.[13]

As a result, understanding exactly what causes auditory hallucinations is not as easy as you might think. There may be several different "mechanisms" our brains use to produce auditory hallucinations. For example, what causes one person to hear tinnitus sounds may be different from what causes the same person to hear musical hallucinations. What causes a hard of hearing person to hear phantom music may be different from what causes a hearing person to hear similar phantom music. What causes a person to hear voice-like sounds may be different from what causes a person to hear music-like sounds.

Because there are so many variables, researchers have come up with a number of theories regarding auditory hallucinations. Any one of them may be the correct explanation, depending on the exact situation.

For example, some research suggests infections of the brain, such as syphilis and Lyme disease can trigger musical

[12] Gurwood, 2003. p. 40.
[13] Hain, ~2002. p. 2.

hallucinations by inflaming parts of the brain. Curing these diseases sometimes cures the hallucinations as well.[14] This accounts for a few of the many cases of auditory hallucinations.

Another theory assumes that something disrupts the normal flow of communication between different parts of the brain. This disruption supposedly causes auditory hallucinations by limiting the function of neurons that normally stop the brain from hallucinating.[15]

However, the most popular theory to explain why so many hard of hearing people experience auditory hallucinations is the theory of sensory deprivation. It centers around the idea that our brains must maintain a certain minimal amount of auditory stimulation from our ears in order to prevent memory traces within our brains from taking over.

When a person loses much of his hearing, such that it falls below this threshold, he may begin to hear auditory hallucinations because the lack of typical auditory input to the hearing area of the brain's temporal lobe allows those areas to become active on their own.[16] It is thought that the perception-bearing circuits become disinhibited,[17] thereby allowing previous memories to be released into awareness, and thus creating auditory hallucinations.[18]

This theory explains why most people that experience musical hallucinations hear songs and musical tunes they have known in the past, often from early childhood. The reason these songs are dredged out of their memories is likely because they are the most strongly encoded memories, and thus most easily summoned up by their music-perception networks.

Incidentally, a person can hear musical hallucinations every hour of the day without any other distortion of reality. This is because our brains process music through a unique network of neurons. Research has shown that these neurons can go wrong without affecting any other part of the brain.

Dr. Timothy Griffiths, at the Newcastle University Medical School, is trying to unravel the mysteries of musical hallucinations. His understanding is that musical hallucinations in hard of hearing people are related to activity within the neural networks that perceive high-level patterns of sound.[19] This

[14] Zimmer, 2004. p. 3.

[15] Rare Hallucinations Make Music in the Mind, 2000. p. 2.

[16] Edell, 1998. p. 1.

[17] Mikkilineni, 1998. p. 2.

[18] Eizenberg, 1987. p. 3.

[19] Griffiths, 2000. p. 2066.

spontaneous activity lies in an area of the brain usually involved in the normal perception of patterns in segmented sounds.[20]

He was surprised to discover similar brain activity in both normally-hearing people listening to music and in hard of hearing people experiencing musical hallucinations. The main difference between the brain activity in these two groups was that the musical hallucinations didn't activate the primary cortex, the first stop for sound in the brain. When people experience musical hallucinations, they use only the parts of the brain responsible for turning simple sounds into complex music.[21] Here is how he thinks it happens.

When sounds first enter the brains of people with normal hearing, they activate a region near the ears called the primary auditory cortex, which starts processing sounds at their most basic level. This area is involved with the perception of individual sounds. From there, the auditory cortex passes the signals to areas that recognize more complex features of music, such as rhythm, key changes and melody. This is the area of the brain involved with the perception of patterns in segmented sounds. From there the signals are sent to the area for the encoding/ recognition of patterned segmented sounds. This latter area communicates **weakly** with the previous area.

In people that experience musical hallucinations, there is obviously no input from the ears to the brain, thus no input or output from the area for the perception of individual sounds. Instead, the area for the perception of patterns in segmented sounds **generates some spontaneous activity** of its own that goes to the area responsible for encoding/recognition of patterned segmented sounds. Unlike in people who do not hear hallucinations, this latter area communicates **strongly** with the previous area. This seems to sustain these hallucinations.[22]

Another way of looking at Griffiths' theory is that the music-processing regions of the brain are continually looking for patterns in the signals arriving from the ears. As these regions recognize a tune, they amplify certain sounds that fit the music and minimize extraneous sounds. However, when no sound is coming into the ears, as is often the case with hard of hearing people, neurons in the music network sometimes spontaneously fire off random impulses. The brain seizes on these signals and tries to impose some structure to them, rummaging though its

[20] Griffiths, 2000. p. 2075.

[21] Zimmer, 2004. pp. 2-3.

[22] Griffiths, 2000. p. 2074.

memory banks for a match. A few notes may suddenly turn into a familiar melody.

For people with normal hearing, these signals may produce a song that is hard to get out of their heads. However, with a constant stream of sounds coming in from their ears, their brains quickly suppress this false music. In the case of hard of hearing people, however, hearing loss cuts off much of this constant stream of sounds, and in some hard of hearing people, their music-seeking circuits go into overdrive. As a result, they hear this phantom music all the time. It seems as real as any normal sound.[23]

The good news is that when hard of hearing people wear hearing aids, and thus receive adequate sound stimulation, they can often suppress these "free-wheeling" musical circuits. As a result, their auditory hallucinations often simply fade into the background.

[23] Zimmer, 2004. p. 3.

Chapter 5

What's in a Name?

The Fear Factor

Just to be told they are experiencing hallucinations scares the wits out of many people because they now think they are crazy. As a result, few people admit to experiencing auditory hallucinations. If they ever do hear phantom sounds, they often try to rationalize away these auditory hallucinations, or put their strange hallucinations into some sort of logical context—no matter how weird that may sound. For example, "Tonya" explained:

> I have been at my wits end with this noise/music in my ear/head. I knew it wasn't tinnitus, and I knew I am not a schizophrenic. I thought maybe I'm getting my hearing back. What a joke! Then I started thinking maybe it's in the **other dimension**, or **aliens**.

"Gretchen" wrote:

> I have been hearing phantom music for the last 2 or 3 months. The music usually sounds like a marching band. I initially thought that I was having some sort of **spiritual experience**.

After surgery for a cochlear implant, "Ashleigh" came up with a novel explanation for her resulting auditory hallucinations. She wrote:

> I had thought maybe they **put some sort of music or something inside the cochlear implant** to keep the hair cells alive before you are hooked up. It was my way of thinking.

Gladys rationalized her phantom sounds as coming from her teeth. She explains:

When I first started having tinnitus in my 20s, **I thought I was picking up some sort of radio signals on my dental bridge!** That was the only context I had for the tones I was experiencing.

Part of the reason accurate statistics on non-psychiatric auditory hallucinations are so hard to come by is that people experiencing auditory hallucinations fear being thought crazy, not only by their doctors, family and friends, but even by their own spouses. Roger explains:

My wife thought I was schizophrenic. I haven't mentioned it since, but my phantom music is still there.

Laurie writes:

My dad admitted to hearing music last night, but while giggling as though he thought anyone might think he was nuts. He was embarrassed.

Gail reports:

For over a year my father has experienced hearing music and voices. He actually copes very well with the sounds, although he says, "if I describe this to most people, **they would think I was crazy.**" He was **reluctant to talk to our family doctor,** but they have all been understanding.

Lorene says:

I was afraid I was going nuts when I thought I was hearing things in my head after my CI surgery. I remember on the morning after the surgery, I was hearing what sounded like some music from a radio. I heard that every day from my surgery until I was hooked up. It almost drove me nuts. Yet, **I never said one word to anyone** about it because **I didn't want them to think I was crazy. I never even said a word to my mom.**

Vera explains:

I pulled up your site and much to my surprise, I found that I am not nuts. **All my family believe I am nuts** because I told them I hear music every waking moment. My music is very real and I hear the entire song. Sometimes over and over and over. I am hard of hearing and wear a hearing aid sometimes.

Loretta writes:

My mother recently began hearing musical auditory hallucinations. We've been to a neurologist and checked out ok. I'm very concerned about her. She is getting very depressed about the noises. **She thinks she is going crazy.**

Roberta's mom also thinks she is going crazy. Roberta explains:

My mother experiences auditory hallucinations. She hears music almost constantly at different sound levels. She is in her mid 80s and was as upset about hearing the music as she was by **the thought that she was going crazy.**

Martha told me:

I have been hearing humming music in my head for over 8 years, and it has gotten progressively worse. **I said nothing** to anybody about this problem until recently because **I was convinced I was going mentally berserk.**

Astrid declared:

I **never** mentioned hearing this auditory hallucination to any doctor because **auditory hallucinations are linked to psychiatric disorders.**

It should be obvious by now that although many people experience auditory hallucinations, most keep this to themselves because, to them, hearing auditory hallucinations is proof that they are crazy.

How Common Are Auditory Hallucinations?

How many people experience auditory hallucinations? The short answer is, "At this point, no one really knows because people **very seldom** admit to hearing auditory hallucinations for **fear of being thought crazy.**" Thus, the occurrence of auditory hallucinations is more common than people generally recognize.[1]

Another obstacle to getting accurate statistics is that most researchers/writers lump both psychiatric and non-psychiatric hallucinations together when they talk about auditory hallucinations. This makes it difficult to obtain reliable statistics on just the people who experience non-psychiatric auditory hallucinations.

Although incidence figures are sketchy at best, there are a number of clues that indicate just how common experiencing auditory hallucinations must be.

[1] Eizenberg, 1987. p. 4.

For example, since I placed my article on auditory hallucinations on the hearinglosshelp.com website, I have received numerous emails from people around the world as the stories on these pages attest. This, alone, reveals that hearing auditory hallucinations is not as rare as you might think. In fact, it is quite a common, though seldom talked about, phenomenon.

One study disclosed that about 12% of the general population have experienced auditory hallucinations. In another study of patients admitted to a medical ward, 32% (16 of 50) of the patients reported experiencing an auditory hallucination at some time in their lives.[2]

In yet another study of 125 people over age 65, 33% of them heard auditory hallucinations. Of those hearing various phantom sounds, 95% heard tinnitus sounds, 2.5% heard phantom voices and another 2.5% heard music that was not there. The author concluded that auditory hallucinations are frequent in elderly hard of hearing people.[3]

We can also draw some conclusions by extrapolating from the incidence figures in people with visual problems who experience visual hallucinations. These visual hallucinations are known as Charles Bonnet syndrome, and are the visual counterpart of non-psychiatric auditory hallucinations. The incidence of Charles Bonnet syndrome in people with low vision in one ophthalmology clinic was 11%.[4] Another researcher reported, "Its prevalence in patients with visual impairments varies from 10% to 15%."[5]

Since auditory hallucinations are supposedly much more common than visual hallucinations,[6] we can assume that the comparable figures for auditory hallucinations are at least this high and likely even higher.

I have confirmed this from my own experience. When I speak to groups of hard of hearing people, I sometimes ask how many have heard such auditory hallucinations and invariably 10% to 30% of the people present feel brave enough to put up their hands.

[2] Eizenberg, 1987. p. 3.

[3] Cole, 2002. p. 1.

[4] Thorpe, 1997. p 24s.

[5] Jacob, 2004. p. 3.

[6] Eizenberg, 1987. p. 3.

You Are Not Crazy

People need to get over the idea that experiencing non-psychiatric auditory hallucinations is a sign of mental illness, instead of it just being a sign something not working quite right in the auditory system. Unfortunately, to the average person, hearing auditory hallucinations is synonymous with "hearing voices" and mental illness, even though the vast majority of phantom sounds have nothing whatsoever to do with mental illness.

Here is an example to illustrate this point. Charles explained to me that his ears were working normally when he walked into the garage where his car was being serviced. However, when he came out a short time later, he was hearing loud phantom sounds. He writes:

> I recently was waiting in an auto garage when the metal plates on the alignment rack I was close to slammed down as a car was being driven off of it.

Voilà, the unexpected loud noise produced instant tinnitus in Charles' head. Is Charles mentally ill because he now hears the constant phantom sounds of tinnitus, itself a type of auditory hallucination? Of course not! Something in his auditory system changed to be sure, but he did not suddenly become mentally ill. Exactly the same principle holds true for people who begin hearing the voices, music and other sounds of non-psychiatric auditory hallucinations.

Furthermore, people who experience Phantom Limb syndrome are not considered crazy even though they "feel" a limb that is no longer there. Neither are people crazy who experience visual hallucinations (Charles Bonnet syndrome), so why should we think it would be any different for people who experience non-psychiatric auditory hallucinations?

In all of these cases, it's because the parts of the brain that process the inputs from these limbs/senses are still active, even though a limb is missing or the sense organ isn't working well any more. This just gives rise to phantom sensations, not psychotic delusions.

The Need for a New Name—Musical Ear Syndrome

Although the nature of non-psychiatric auditory hallucinations is not psychotic, the presumed association between auditory hallucinations and mental illness is strongly entrenched in most people's minds. In fact, the general public automatically equates anything with the name "hallucination" in it with mental illness.

Notice that all the names used to describe this condition—auditory hallucinations, pseudo-auditory hallucinations, psychological auditory hallucinations, non-pathologic auditory hallucinations, musical hallucinations, non-psychiatric auditory hallucinations—all contain the word "hallucinations." Upon hearing any of these terms, the average person instantly forms a mental image of a crazy person.

We need a name that doesn't have the negative connotations associated with the word "hallucinations." Apart from the above names, there are a couple of existing possibilities. One is the word **paracusis**, the other is the term **auditory imagery**.

Paracusis is rarely used to describe auditory hallucinations. According to *Stedman's Medical Dictionary*, paracusis is defined as either "impaired hearing" or "auditory illusions or hallucinations."[7] Paracusis comes from the Greek "para" meaning "near," thus denoting a departure from the normal, and "akousis," the Greek word for "hearing."

Paracusis is, therefore, anything that departs from normal hearing. It seems to be used mostly for describing distorted hearing rather than auditory hallucinations. For example, with paracusis, sound volumes may be altered, changed in tone or timbre, or may even sound strange and disagreeable.[8]

Since paracusis is more commonly used to describe distorted hearing and is seldom used to describe auditory hallucinations, this name would be confusing at best.

In Great Britain, some professionals use the term **auditory imagery** as a synonym for musical hallucinations. For example, "some people hear their tinnitus as music or songs instead of the usual sounds. These are called 'musical hallucinations' or 'auditory imagery.'"[9]

[7] Stedman's Medical Dictionary, 2000. p. 1309.

[8] Troost, ~2003. p. 3.

[9] Musical Hallucinations, 2003. p. 1.

This term, too, is confusing as mental health professionals in the USA **use the same term to mean something entirely different**, and even contrast auditory imagery with auditory hallucinations, showing that they are two different things. For example, psychiatrist Dr. David Silbersweig "discusses how hearing auditory hallucinations differs from things like dreaming and auditory imagery (i.e., being able to conjure up someone's voice in your mind) in people without schizophrenia."[10] Inasmuch as auditory imagery is really nothing more than remembering what something sounded like, it obviously cannot be the same thing as hearing auditory hallucinations.

Since both paracusis and auditory imagery are used to describe other conditions and thus would confuse people, and since all the other terms in use today contain the word "hallucinations" and the negative connotations that go with it, it is obvious that there needs to be a new name to describe non-psychiatric auditory hallucinations—a name that doesn't even convey a subliminal message that a person with this condition might be mentally ill.

Since the vast majority of people who experience non-psychiatric auditory hallucinations hear some sort of phantom musical sounds, I am hereby naming this condition "Musical Ear syndrome" (MES). I define Musical Ear syndrome as:

> **Musical Ear Syndrome (MES)**: Hearing phantom sounds (auditory hallucinations) of a non-psychiatric nature, often musical, but also including voices and other associated sounds, commonly found in, but not limited to, elderly, hard of hearing people with tinnitus who lack adequate sound stimulation.

I am hoping that by using a name that has no negative connotations (and one that even sounds like it might be something desirable to have) that the stigma of hearing non-psychiatric phantom sounds will fade away.

In the remainder of this book, I use the terms "non-psychiatric auditory hallucinations," "auditory hallucinations," "Musical Ear syndrome" and its abbreviation "MES" interchangeably.

---

[10] Haahr, 2004. p. 3.

Chapter 6

Understanding Musical Ear Syndrome

Musical Ear Syndrome Symptoms

Musical Ear syndrome (MES), as its name implies, is comprised of a number of symptoms, which, when taken together, form a syndrome. Typically, but not always, there is a constellation of 5 symptoms that seem to predispose people to hearing such phantom sounds. These symptoms include:

1. Often the person is **elderly**.

2. Generally, the person is **hard of hearing**.

3. Often the person lacks adequate **auditory stimulation**.

4. Almost always the person has **tinnitus**.

5. Often the person is either **anxious**, **stressed** or **depressed**.

In addition, typically the people reporting hearing such sounds are **female**.

A person does not have to exhibit all 5 symptoms in order to have Musical Ear syndrome, but many people with MES exhibit 3 or more of the above symptoms. For as yet unknown reasons, there are people that prove to be exceptions to this rule. Perhaps, in the future, researchers will discover why.

Not Limited to Elderly People

Although Musical Ear syndrome is more-commonly experienced by seniors, these phantom sounds are not limited to elderly people by any means. Such hallucinations occur in younger adults too when they lose their hearing. Here is Melanie's experience.

> I've had a progressive hearing loss due to otosclerosis over the past 16 years. I functioned quite well for most of that time by wearing hearing aids. Suddenly, on June 6th, in a span of about 20 minutes I lost just about all of my sensorineural hearing and became deaf.
>
> Since that time I not only have my usual loud tinnitus, but also ever-increasing auditory hallucinations! It seems that my brain just can't stand to not hear, so it's filling my head with all sorts of sounds. At the moment I have a repertoire of at least 25 different "tracks" that play over and over again, although usually only 4 or 5 are playing at any given time (plus the ringing from tinnitus).
>
> My different musical tracks all have variations that come and go— some reverberating, some hummed in rounds, different instruments taking over the same refrains, etc. I seem to get something new every day!

Some children also experience auditory hallucinations. Paula writes:

> My 10 year old daughter tells me she has started hearing noises and voices and naturally this scares me. Prior to this, she has told me she believes her hearing is impaired as she has to ask people to repeat themselves. Last week was the first time she told me she heard voices—division problems—numbers. Last night she was sitting at the computer and said she heard a scream and this morning while she was taking a shower, she heard wowowowowowowow—wow being repeated. At this time, she is congested and taking *Dimetapp* for her nose.

(In this girl's case, her auditory hallucinations may have been caused by the flu/cold she was experiencing and/or the *Dimetapp* she was taking. *Dimetapp* contains **Pseudoephedrine**. One of the rare side effects of **Pseudoephedrine** is hallucinations.)

Not Limited to Hard of Hearing People

The vast majority of the people who experience auditory hallucinations also have a significant hearing loss. However, for whatever reason, some people with normal hearing also hear these phantom sounds. Amethyst asks:

> I hear what sounds like a radio in my head, only **I'm not hard of hearing at all**. Am I going crazy?

Diana explains:

I hear orchestral music most any time it's quiet, which is usually late in the evening and through the wee hours. I hear fuzzy bursts that sound to me like words, at least the inflection and pacing of words or even names, but I can't quite make them out. Now the odd thing is, **I have phenomenal hearing**.

Carol reports:

I have no history of hearing loss. Yet, for the past few years I have experienced the unbidden music, identifiable and repetitive (complete with applause!) on a sporadic basis. I really thought I had a neighbor with an endless affection for the *Battle Hymn of the Republic*. I continue to hear the music since outside sounds don't always mask it.

Not Limited to Women

Often the literature reports auditory hallucinations are much more commonly found in women than in men,[1] as though being female was somehow a predisposing factor. Being female has nothing to do with hearing auditory hallucinations, even though 70% to 80% of the reports of musical hallucinations come from women.[2]

From my own experience, I also have found that 75% of the people contacting me about their auditory hallucinations have been women. In addition, women contacted me 7% of the time on behalf of their elderly fathers/fathers-in-law. Men accounted for just 18%.

Thus, at first glance, it appears that women are much more likely to experience auditory hallucinations than men. However, I believe these figures are grossly misleading. I believe that the true likelihood of people hearing auditory hallucinations is about equal between the sexes. Let me explain.

During the 1990s, I discovered that about 80% of the attendees at our hearing loss coping skills classes being held in western Canada were women. This was surprising since more men than women have hearing losses. It is also interesting that this 80% figure corresponds almost exactly with the percentage of women seeking help for their auditory hallucinations. Why?

It appears the main reason for this is that far more women than men are willing to speak up and seek help for their auditory

[1] Thorpe, 1997. p 25s.

[2] Folmer, 2002. pp. 1-2.

hallucinations, just like they do when they have hearing losses or other medical conditions. As a result, the incidence figures are quite skewed in favor of women.

In addition, since women typically live longer than men, many women end up as widows. When this happens, they typically live alone in quiet environments—another factor in hearing auditory hallucinations.

Definition of Auditory Hallucinations

The definition of an auditory hallucination (psychiatric or otherwise) includes three parts.

1. It occurs in the absence of a sound stimulus. In other words, it is a phantom sound.

2. It has the full force or impact of a real sound. In other words, you can't tell it apart from a real sound.

3. It is not under your direct and voluntary control. In other words, nothing you consciously do or say will make it stop.[3]

Although this definition may be true for people who hear psychiatric auditory hallucinations, it often breaks down when describing people who have Musical Ear syndrome.

For example, although non-psychiatric auditory hallucinations generally occur in the absence of a sound stimulus, sometimes a continuous sound stimulus may trigger musical hallucinations in some people, such as flying in a plane. (See the section "Constant Background Noise" in Chapter 7.)

Furthermore, initially a person hearing auditory hallucinations may not be able to distinguish between reality and their hallucinations, but they soon/eventually learn which is which. Of course, hard of hearing people can be (and are) fooled too. (See the section "Pseudo-Auditory Hallucinations" in Chapter 3.)

Finally, although non-psychiatric auditory hallucinations are not generally amenable to direct control, some people are able to impose their will to some degree on their hallucinations. (See next section.)

[3] Fadirepo, ~2002. p. 3.

Generally Not Under a Person's Conscious Control

Auditory hallucinations are generally not under a person's conscious control. For example, Roger found that he could not stop or influence his auditory hallucinations. He reported:

I tested this by doing things that would distract me, even humming or singing other melodies, but **it kept on by itself**.

Here is "Mindy's" experience. She explains:

I hear the same few songs over and over again. I have said out loud, **"Stop it!"** when the music really gets on my nerves. If anyone heard me they surely would think I am crazy. And **saying that does not make it stop**.

Diana writes:

I cannot change the tunes I hear. I thought maybe if I was making this stuff up in my head that I could direct it or refine it into something I know. **Doesn't work**. Whatever is playing **is** playing.

"Justin's" auditory hallucinations reappear right in the middle of a tune as he becomes aware of them after being distracted by other sounds. There is nothing he can do about them. He reports:

My musical hallucinations appear to play in the background all of the time, independent of what I am doing. It doesn't prevent any activities. I can become involved in activities and forget about it. However, as soon as these activities cease the music reappears in the middle of some tune. The reappearance is unexpected because I am not thinking about the music in any way whatsoever. The tune is different from the one that I ceased to hear when I began the activity. The music appears to switch from background to foreground whenever the outside sound has low volume. For example, I am now sitting alone at the computer and can hear it quite clearly. I can talk aloud to myself and still hear the tune in the background.

"Heather" relates:

The last 3 days my mom keeps hearing *Silent Night* and *Oh Come All Ye Faithful* over and over again. **She has tried to make it go away, but can't**.

Ernestine writes:

I tried singing a lullaby out loud in hopes the "phantom" would pick it up but **so far no luck**.

Chris explains:

I can purposefully "sing" a song in my head, but **it doesn't change the music I'm "hearing"**.

Some People Have Limited Control

Although most people cannot control their auditory hallucinations in any way, some people have had limited success in controlling theirs. For example, although Chris said (above), "it doesn't change the music I'm hearing," this didn't stop her from trying to manipulate her auditory hallucinations. She continues:

I have auditory hallucinations so real that **I've tried to manipulate them** just to have some fun.

After trying for a month, she finally succeeded in gaining a bit of control over her musical hallucinations. She relates:

I can now "request" a song and most of the time it works—but not always. As I become more exploratory (and perhaps more accepting) the songs become more pliable. Sometimes I can say "stop it" and they fade away little by little.

A few other people, like Chris, seem to have some degree of control over their phantom music—at least part of the time. Patty explains:

I hear sounds like what I call "the vampires are coming" music—from old movies—an organ would be playing. I also hear many recognizable hymns. **I can change the hymns at will or change the key**. I am not a schizophrenic and am not on any medications. I have moderate hearing loss and tinnitus.

At times, some people can change their hallucinations temporarily. "Tony" writes:

My wife heard *Silent Night* sung by a very good choir of mostly men. A day later she heard the *Vienna Waltz* over and over again. **At times she could change the songs temporarily**.

Love Them or Hate Them

Some people can't stand their auditory hallucinations. Others really enjoy hearing them, while still others have a love/hate relationship with theirs.

Annoying Auditory Hallucinations

For many people, their auditory hallucinations are definitely annoying. One researcher declares: "**All** the people who experience such hallucinations with whom I've talked—describe symptoms that are persistent, vivid, loud, localized somewhere in real space, outside their control, and **definitely annoying**."[4]

Auditory hallucinations can be annoying—especially when they interrupt sleep. Igor explains:

I find auditory hallucinations **annoying** because they repeat themselves without stop at any time of the day or night—but they mostly occur at night. Sometimes during the night they **prevent me from getting a good sleep**. I hear music. It is like a band with saxophones and probably trumpets playing a fast tune. These sounds never completely disappear.

Enjoyable Auditory Hallucinations

Not everyone finds their auditory hallucinations annoying, however. In fact, a good number of people enjoy their musical hallucinations. Diana declares:

I do **enjoy** the [phantom] music.

Anita writes:

My mom is hearing music (mostly classical music and all music that she likes) and has recently come to understand that no one else can hear this music. She rather **enjoys** it.

Malisa goes even further, She loves what she hears.

I **love** my phantom voices. I use my phantom voices and music to entertain myself.

Once she realized what was happening, Marcy began to enjoy her phantom music too. She recounted:

The first song I heard was *America the Beautiful*, followed by *Amazing Grace*. Since then, I've had it almost constantly while awake for the last 7 days, with about 6 different general tunes. On the lighter side, **"How does one expand the repertoire?"**

Jane, who has normal hearing, yet hears phantom music, explains:

For years I've been "hearing" music of various sorts when I lay in bed waiting to go to sleep—a wide variety, from band and orchestral, to

[4] Deutsch, 2002. p. 1.

Irish folk music, symphony, opera and so on. **The music itself is really quite pleasant** most of the time, except when the triumphant, flourishing finales get too frequent and out of hand.

"Gretchen" writes:

I have been hearing [phantom] music for the last 2 or 3 months. The music usually sounds like a marching band. Sometimes I hear different sections of a marching band (tuba, trumpets, etc). I find the music **very pleasing** (especially when it sounds celestial).

Love/Hate Relationship with Auditory Hallucinations

Some people have sort of a love/hate relationship with their auditory hallucinations. Mary Lou writes:

I have so many auditory hallucinations sometimes it drives me crazy. I swear sometimes people are talking in another room. On the other hand, it also keeps me company. I cannot make out what the voices say, but **I am still glad they're there**.

Martha explains:

I have been hearing humming music in my head for over 8 years. I hear the humming of different songs (no words). Sometimes Christmas carols, sometimes hymns, sometimes just songs that come from nowhere. Usually I am hearing a repeat of just one stanza of a song, not the whole song. There are times that the repeats get quite fast, over and over and over. It is at this particular time that I feel like it could really get on my nerves.

Broad Range of Experiences

The experiences of people with Musical Ear syndrome seem almost endless. Some aspects of MES are common to many people. However, as the following stories demonstrate, no two people's experiences are exactly the same.

Great Variety of Music, Tunes and Other Sounds

Auditory hallucinations often consist of continuous, repetitive, familiar tunes, with or without words. They may range from simple tunes to orchestral music. Some people experience different songs and types of music each time. Others hear the same music every time.

The type of music heard varies widely from country to country. For example, a French person heard popular French chansons, another person heard Mozart while a Canadian heard Glenn Miller big band music.[5] Australians often hear *"Waltzing Matilda"* while Americans hear *"The Star Spangled Banner."*

"Audrey" has experienced Musical Ear syndrome for some years. She hears all sorts of music—choral singing, soloists, orchestral music and occasionally more like someone calling her name. It's intermittent, any time of day or night, any situation. She is very hard of hearing and wears hearing aids.[6]

Michelle's repertoire of songs is more limited. She writes:

I am 47 and wear one hearing aid. I hear music that isn't even playing in the house like *The Star Spangled Banner*, or *America the Beautiful*, or Elvis Presley. The word are very clear and the tune is also.

"Sheila" only hears one song. She explains:

The only tune I ever get is *Waltzing Matilda* as if it were being played on the bells of an ice-cream van.[7]

"Dallas," describing his auditory hallucinations, said:

I had real life sounds like a jet airplane taking off, or someone talking, or classical music.

Dori asks:

Has anyone ever heard marching songs? I used to hear them so much I would actually start marching sometimes!

Diana writes:

My auditory hallucinations usually take the form of a song I last heard. Right now it is *Thank You for the Music* by Abba. Nice song but it gets old after hearing it continuously for 24 hrs!

Sometimes Linda's auditory hallucinations latch onto some real sounds. She explains:

I just came out of the beauty supply store. They had a great big artificial Santa singing *Jingle Bells* very loudly. Now, my "tinnitus" is singing it too and it's driving me nuts.

Melanie hears quite a repertoire of sounds. She told me:

My auditory hallucinations include everything from several different musical refrains (mostly hummed by a men's choir, but also played by violin), water dripping, plates clattering, dogs barking, the sound of a radio playing with a D.J. talking (undecipherable), slowed down

[5] Scans uncover "Music of the Mind," 2000. p. 2.

[6] RNID Discussion Forum, 2004. pp. 1-2.

[7] RNID Discussion Forum, 2004. p. 2.

voices (also undecipherable), the sound of a Siberian wind swirling, car horns honking, sirens, the tape I've named *Swamp Animals at Sunset*, a Native American chant, rainfall, a South American pan pipe (flute)—the list goes on and on.

Allan writes:

I also experience occasional sounds that are not there. Usually gongs or bells but occasionally a shouted word. I had this quite a bit when my hearing loss went from moderate to more severe.

"Tonya" hears weird and somewhat scary sounds. She relates:

I have been at my wits end with this noise/music in my ear/head. My phantom noises started around 10 years ago with a sound of bomb alarms (ones you hear in old war movies). It went on for about a year or two, and I haven't heard it since. Also, about 10 years ago, I used to hear someone call my name, but it wasn't happening enough to be concerned about.

Ones that scared me most started about 3-4 years ago. I heard "NO!" and shortly after I heard "BOO!", only few minutes apart. Music and choir sounds became prevalent shortly after this. The music and sounds are usually erratic and unusual. I seldom find any rhythm or recognition, as they are rarely anything like the ones we hear around us. However, I do hear the same ones repeatedly. I have three or four regular sounds/noises and several odd ones (wind howling, screaming sounds, etc).

Gail's father hears a bunch of different "radio" sounds. She reports:

My father is 88 and has suffered from tinnitus for years. He uses hearing aids. His hearing is pretty bad. For over a year he has experienced hearing music or voices (sporting events, etc.) at various times of the day. If he plays music he can drown them out.

The music is very understandable, as are the voices. For quite some time he thought he was hearing someone's radio outside his window, playing music that he didn't typically listen to; country, opera, etc. He would also "hear" a ball game being announced, but not an old familiar game or announcer. The voice might be something like an auctioneer, or someone repeating a numeral.

Here is Dot's experience with MES. She explains:

I noticed my hearing failing about 8 years ago and have worn a hearing aid for about 6 years. I have just turned 78. I can hear phantom music playing all the time. The sounds seem to be coming from behind me or at the right side at some distance.

Schubert's Ghost

Musical Ear syndrome has been around for a long time. Composer Robert Schumann also heard auditory hallucinations toward the end of his life. At night, he heard musical notes and believed that he heard an angelic choir singing to him. He also heard the music of Beethoven and Schubert. He jotted down the music in February, 1854 and called it the *Theme* (WoO, 1854).[8] He said he was taking dictation from Schubert's ghost.[9]

[8] Lindsay, 2003. p. 1.

[9] Zimmer, 2004. p. 2.

I first noticed the music which sounded like *Amazing Grace* just before Christmas only in a certain eating place and thought it was background music or carols. I was not aware of it at any other time but noticed it when I went to that particular place a few weeks later. I asked my friend if she could hear it, which, of course, she denied. I gradually realized it was with me all the time.

It is definitely musical and reminds me of an old-fashioned organ. At one stage, when intermingled with other noises and music, it sounded like the full version of *Amazing Grace* over and over again. It really is a pleasant soothing rhythm. Sometimes it sounds like *Silent Night*. When I wake in the morning, it is very soft and takes 5 minutes or so before I can really hear it.

The tune has developed into more or less the same phrase for about six times then it varies. Sometimes it is quiet, other times louder, sometimes faster, sometimes monotonous for a longer time before it changes key. It annoys me at times especially at the films when there is no conversation or it intermingles with soft music.

Just before Christmas it sounded very "Christmassy" with a nice slow *Silent Night* and *Amazing Grace*, but now the same bar goes on for much longer before it changes key and expands the tune more to a bright cheery tune, but certainly not a recognizable one.

Madhuri, writing about her mom, reports:

My mom recently lost her hearing in her right hear. She was initially able to hear what could be diagnosed as tinnitus. Now, one month past the episode, she mentions time and again of being able to hear music in her ears—sometimes prayers to god by a group, led by a male voice, and at other times, like listening to a tape recorder or the same song (a few old movie songs—mostly by a male voice), again and again.

How to get her to stop hearing this? As long as she is hearing this music, it takes her twice as much effort to listen to what we say.

Marie recounts:

I occasionally wake up in the morning to what sounds like people talking outside my window or a radio being played loudly. However, I can't discriminate the words. Without my hearing aids in, I hear nothing unless it's a very loud noise.

Ernestine declares:

I hear the beginning of *Around the World in 80 Days* and *The Star Spangled Banner* and *Reveille* and *Taps* and several repetitive notes, and some songs I only recognize vaguely.

I've co-existed with common tinnitus ever since I can remember—steam hissing, subway trains, and a waterfall (Niagara)—always there but at least it's steady and doesn't demand my attention.

I wish I understood how the musical program is selected, whether it's random and why it totally ignores my taste. Most of my phantom music is military and I'm totally unmilitary.

The phantom music now repeats the same piece that has a lot of flourishes but little melody and is loudest all night and whenever I try to sleep.

Often Religious or Patriotic Songs

One intriguing aspect of many MES experiences is that they are generally religious or patriotic in nature. For example, "Andrew" hears both patriotic and religious songs. He writes:

A few weeks ago I was sitting at home alone when I began to hear music which appeared to be associated with my right ear. The music was **mostly simple songs such as patriotic tunes or religious songs, but sometimes a few bars of classical music**. A tune repeats itself for a while and then changes to another.

"Rachel" heard what sounded like *The Star Spangled Banner* playing over and over in her head. She wrote:

I don't have screaming tinnitus—just auditory hallucinations. Here I am thinking that hearing *The Star Spangled Banner* playing in my head was just normal tinnitus. Songs, songs, songs, but mainly *The Star Spangled Banner*.

Seasonal Quality to the Music

Quite often auditory hallucinations take on a seasonal quality. Thus, Christmas carols are commonly heard during the winter season. For example, "Sharon" wrote:

My 66 year old mom lost 95% of her hearing in her left ear 25 years ago. She lost almost all of the rest in both ears 2 months ago. The last 3 days (this was written December 28th) she keeps hearing *Silent Night* and *Oh Come All Ye Faithful* over and over again. It gets so loud that she can't sleep. She says that it is beautiful singing with a full orchestra, but would really like some sleep.

In another example, Susan writes:

It was just after Thanksgiving when I became rather suddenly totally deaf. I kept hearing 2 or 3 Christmas carols and one Chanukah song over and over. It was pleasant but I was afraid if it continued too long

I would get very annoyed by it. After the holiday season the songs changed, and then totally disappeared. It probably lasted about 10-12 weeks.

Ed's wife also heard Christmas music around Christmas. He explains:

My wife hears the same song being sung over and over in her head. The music started a few days before Christmas. The first song was *Silent Night* sung by a very good choir of mostly men. It came in quite loud. A day later it was the *Vienna Waltz* over and over again so clear it was like being at a musical production.

Often Songs Learned in Childhood

The songs many elderly hard of hearing people "hear" are often familiar tunes they remember from when they were children. Perhaps they heard this kind of music in childhood more often than other types of music.[10]

For example, one hard of hearing elderly woman heard old forms of German hymns dating back to when she was a girl in a German-speaking area of Russia. Interestingly enough, she had not spoken German regularly for close to 60 years. Another person heard Italian opera that her parents used to listen to. Still others hear hymns, sea shanties, jazz or pop tunes.[11]

Unusual Experiences with Musical Ear Syndrome

One unusual experience is where a person hears her own voice repeated as an auditory hallucination. Frank writes:

My cousin, Shirley has experienced auditory hallucinations. The problem manifests itself mainly as repetitive music, but also **occasionally as repetition of her own spoken sentences from conversation**.

Malisa also has had a very unusual experience with Musical Ear syndrome as her hearing deteriorated. Here is how she described hers:

I hear single musical tones—clear as can be that would ring for a day or maybe two, then would stop, never to be heard again. I started charting them on music paper for each ear. I've watched me going deaf one note at a time, like candles burning out. I'm down to the very, very bass notes on the piano. Hopefully they'll hold for a little while longer. (The only place I have any measurable hearing is in the 250 and 500 Hz. range at 80-90 dB).

[10] Deutsch, 2002. p. 2.
[11] Zimmer, 2004. p. 2.

Chapter 7

Causes of Musical Ear Syndrome

Auditory hallucinations may arise from several causes—some organic (e.g. regional brain atrophy, brain damage, infectious diseases, drugs) and some functional (depression, anxiety). Sometimes, doctors err when they seek to make their diagnosis as either organic or functional when, in fact, both kinds may be present.[1] In addition, a person may even experience both psychiatric and non-psychiatric auditory hallucinations at the same time.

Studies have linked auditory hallucinations to a range of things including old age, hearing loss, brain tumors, drug overdoses and even liver transplants.[2]

Following are a number of the more common causes of auditory hallucinations. Some are organic and some are functional. This gives an indication of the broad range of factors that can cause auditory hallucinations in perfectly sane people.

1. Hearing Loss/Lack of Auditory Stimulation

Hallucinations can occur as a result of reduced sensory stimulation. Doctors call this sensory deprivation. Thus, people (especially hard of hearing people) may experience auditory hallucinations due to sensory deprivation in situations where they hear few environmental sounds.[3] Proof of this is that people hear auditory hallucinations more often when it is quiet than when it is noisy.[4]

Likewise, people suffering from chronic and extensive hearing loss more commonly hear hallucinations than people with

[1] Eizenberg, 1987. p. 4.

[2] Zimmer, 2004. p. 2.

[3] Schielke, 2000. p. 2.

[4] Fadirepo, ~2002. p. 10.

normal hearing. Researchers think that their long-term auditory sensory deprivation leads to a release of musical and other memories.[5] Thus, when a hard of hearing person's brain feels the loss of auditory input, it sometimes decides to dredge up old memories, and uses them to manufacture music and other sounds of its own. In fact, researchers have discovered that auditory hallucinations typically increase in people with progressive hearing loss.[6]

Made Worse by Silence

Auditory hallucinations caused by sensory deprivation are particularly noticeable when it is very quiet, thus compounding the effects of the hearing loss. Anita writes:

> My mom is 80 and she is losing her hearing. She has tinnitus and has been hearing auditory hallucinations (mostly classical music and other music that she likes) for about 5 months. She has recently come to understand that no one else can hear this music. She lives alone and moved into a new place that is **very quiet** about 5 months ago. Before she moved into this new place, she lived on an active small city street. She did not hear music like this before she moved.

Ken, also hard of hearing, wrote:

> I would often lie half awake in the **quietness** of the early morning and hear a "radio." A guy would be talking like they did in the 50s. Kind of a monotone voice and all the advertisements like they did back then. It always sounded so real.

In these cases, there appears to be a close connection between the hearing loss, the quiet environment and the resulting auditory hallucinations. Typically, the hallucinations are heard the loudest when it is quiet—which normally occurs during the night when a person is in bed.

Here is another example. Keith writes:

> My wife's uncle lives alone in a small semi-detached house. He is blind and has a tremendous loss of hearing. He is 93 years old, and his few pleasures are listening to the television and the radio. But as you can guess, he has to have the volume turned real high in order to listen to it. Unfortunately, **the adjacent neighbor has lately started playing very loud music against his bedroom wall from 1 am to 6 am**, in retaliation I suppose!

Notice that in this case also, the hallucinations are heard when it is quiet. This elderly man is totally fooled by his

[5] Musical Hallucinations Linked to Brain Disorders, 2000. p. 1.

[6] Fadirepo, ~2002. p. 7.

hallucinations and ascribes the loud music he hears to his nasty neighbor retaliating for his playing his radio and TV loud during the day—never dreaming that the music is all in his head.

A moment's reflection reveals that his neighbor wouldn't really do this, or the neighbor wouldn't be able to sleep with all that racket either!

Darlene discovered that the rooms where she hears her auditory hallucinations the most are the two rooms where it is quiet and she is generally alone. She writes:

> I've tried to find out where the music was coming from by walking into other rooms and opening doors and windows. It is most noticeable in two rooms of my house—my bedroom and a spare room with the computer. **These are the rooms where I am alone most of the time**. It usually goes away when I go into the kitchen or living room. It is obviously not coming from outside or downstairs, nor is it the noise of the air conditioner, fans, appliances, etc.

Notice that in her case, when she goes into the kitchen where typically people make more noise, her music goes away. Again, this shows that auditory hallucinations thrive in silent situations.

Bizarre Behavior Can Result from Hearing Auditory Hallucinations

Sometimes people who hear auditory hallucinations seem to have bizarre behavior associated with hearing their phantom sounds. However, their behavior becomes understandable when you realize they are responding rationally and appropriately to the sounds they think they are hearing. Here is an interesting example. Lenore writes:

> We are at out wits end about what to do about my dear 90 year old father-in-law. He has been hard of hearing for some time and it is getting progressively worse. He wears hearing aids. He hears auditory hallucinations. His MRI, EEG and CT scan were all normal. The geriatric psychiatrist tested him and found no dementia. He mainly hears loud music when **alone** in his apartment, oftentimes in the middle of the night. Unfortunately, **he has taken to knocking on the downstairs landlady's door (at 3 A.M.) telling her to turn the music down**. We have been with him a few times when he heard the music—none of us heard anything.

Notice that doctors had thoroughly examined this man and found no traces of mental illness. Thus, they were at a loss to explain his apparently irrational behavior because they were ignorant of Musical Ear syndrome.

Other people actually try to block the phantom sounds they hear by closing the windows in their houses, blocking the chimney, stuffing cotton wool in their ears, or sleeping with a pillow over their heads.[7]

This apparently bizarre and irrational behavior becomes perfectly rational when you realize they are trying to block out what appears to them to be real, intrusive sounds from external sources. They generally stop this behavior when they come to understand they are just hearing phantom sounds.

If you are dealing with apparently irrational behavior due to a person hearing auditory hallucinations, you need to understand two things. First, this music is totally real to the person "hearing" it. Thus, the person hearing such phantom sounds has **no** reason to suspect he is hearing an hallucination. Second, the sounds often seem to have directionality. As a result, the phantom sounds may appear to be coming from another room or even from another building rather than from inside a person's head. Therefore, in the above case, the man's pounding on his landlady's door at 3:00 AM to get her to turn her music off begins to make sense, since, to him, the sounds seem to be coming from her apartment.

Notice another apparently irrational thought this man has. Lenore further explains:

> He thinks the landlady **knows exactly when he lays down to sleep**—of course, **that is when she turns the music all the way up**.

Also, remember the man who thought his neighbor was playing music against his wall to get back at him?

> Unfortunately, **the adjacent neighbor has lately started playing very loud music against his bedroom wall from 1 am to 6 am**, in retaliation I suppose!

Both of these gentlemen had similar irrational thoughts about their neighbors. This happens because in the quietness of the night, these phantom sounds have no competition, so seem ever so much louder. Thus, these men had "rational"

[7] Zimmer, 2004. p. 2.

reasons for believing that someone just turned the music way up when they were trying to go to sleep—even though both were totally wrong in their assumptions.

May Feel Vibrations

There is another fascinating aspect in the case of Lenore's father-in-law. He holds what appears to be another totally irrational belief. Lenore continues:

> My father-in-law also believes his landlady has a **vibrating device or machine that makes the floor vibrate**. Other than this, he is very lucid. His mind and memory are very sharp.

Before you write this man off as crazy, remember, his doctors carried out extensive tests and declared him sane. His apparently irrational thinking is not as weird as it first seems. In fact, one of the stranger things that sometimes happens when a person hears certain auditory hallucinations is that the person not only "hears" these phantom sounds, but, at the same time, may also "feel" the vibrations these sounds seem to produce. Unless you have experienced the sensation of feeling these phantom vibrations, you have no idea just how real these phantom sensations seem.

For example, for several years before I remarried, I lived alone. It was then that I began to notice I'd "hear" a low rumbling sound and at the same time, the floor (or whole house) would start vibrating. My first thought was that there was something wrong with the furnace.

The furnace was old and the fan was not perfectly balanced so it rumbled as it blew air into the plenum. This made the plenum vibrate and thus vibrated the floor—or so I thought. As a result, when this first began to occur, I'd run down to the basement to see what was wrong with the furnace. I'd put my hand on the plenum or the furnace itself since I couldn't hear if the furnace was running or not. I was shocked to discover that there was no vibration whatsoever. The plenum was cold. Neither the furnace nor the fan were even running! It slowly dawned on me that both the sensation of sound and the sensation of the floor vibrating were all in my head.

While I was trying to convince my brain that these "furnace" sensations were all in my head, my brain decided on fool me another way. My brain now produced rumbling sounds and floor vibrations that seemed to come from an 18-wheeler parked outside on the street with its motor idling. I'd look out the windows at both the front and the back of the house but there were no trucks in sight. Then I'd check the furnace again just to be sure. Again, I began to learn that both of these sensations were all in my head. They were phantom sensations—not real sounds and real vibrations.

Now I know that when I "hear" and "feel" these rumbling sensations, it is almost certainly phantom sensations occurring in my head. Unfortunately, elderly people may not be as able to make the connection between the "floor vibrating" and their auditory hallucinations, as was the case of Lenore's father-in-law.

"Feeling" rumbling sensations is not as rare as you might think. It's not just Lenore's father-in-law and me that "feel" such sensations. From talking with numerous elderly hard of hearing people, I've discovered that some of them also have similar experiences. For example, Rose relates:

> I think tinnitus or something similar has struck me with a vengeance. Either that, or I am slowly going out of my mind. Tonight, at about 2 AM, I was awakened by a continuous high piercing **vibrating** sound. I checked the house to see if I could locate something. After about a half hour things seem to have subsided. I am not "hearing" the vibrations any more. I really usually am a sane logical lady and don't know what is happening to me. I live alone, and I am 80 years old.

Dan had a somewhat similar experience. He writes:

> My left ear has an annoying rumbling sound in it. It is not just the sound I hear, but also **I can actually feel the rumbling**.

Carolyn's experiences were very similar to mine. She explains:

> Late at night when I don't have my hearing aids on, I am sure **I hear motors of large trucks** working right outside our bedroom windows. We are the only ones living on our little country lane. There's no traffic of any kind outside my bedroom windows. My husband swears there's no noises at all.

On two other occasions she told me:

> The other night I could not sleep due to my **"hearing" a low rumbling like trucks** were lining up right outside my bedroom window.

and,

I am absolutely sure that there are trucks and bulldozers working just outside my bedroom window late at night when it is quiet. And yes, **I have felt the vibrations! People would think I was going off the deep end if I told anyone that.** I have mentioned it to husband and he'd shake his head slightly in a bit of awe.

Like me, Carolyn now understands that the above sensations are auditory hallucinations. However, to the casual observer, it is so easy to assume that people who "hear" such phantom sounds and feel phantom "vibrations" must be crazy. In actual fact, all of the above people are sane and lucid. They are simply describing some of the strange, and at times scary, auditory hallucinations they have experienced as a result of their Musical Ear syndrome.

2. Drugs

Taking drugs and medications is another major cause of people experiencing auditory hallucinations. Most people know that some "recreational" drugs such as alcohol, lysergic acid diethylamide (LSD), marijuana (Pot), mescaline (Peyote), methamphetamines (Meth) and others can cause auditory hallucinations.[8] However, it seldom crosses the minds of most people that some of the prescription drugs they are taking can also cause such phantom sounds.

Eventually, however, some people start putting two and two together. They begin to wonder if there is a connection between the drugs they are taking and the phantom sounds they are hearing. For example, "Stanley" asks:

I was about to take a nap when I heard the national anthem being played. I went into the next room and asked my wife if they were playing it on TV. No! Well, I continued to hear it for a period of time. Then all of a sudden it went to *Amazing Grace*. Now it is a repetitive three or four notes. **I have just begun taking *Remeron*. Could this be the source?**

It sure could be! In fact, **Mirtazapine** (*Remeron*) is known to cause hallucinations in some people, such as the auditory hallucinations "Stanley" experienced.

"Irene" also wondered whether drugs were causing her mom's musical hallucinations. She questions:

---

[8] Folmer, 2002. p. 1.

My mom has had a hearing loss for many years. This last year she started hearing music and now voices. My mom was put on *Celexa* for anxiety four weeks ago. **Could this have any relation to her problem? It does coincide with her hearing "voices."**

Again, there may be a connection. For example, **Citalopram** (*Celexa*) can cause hallucinations in some people. The fact that this lady began hearing voices soon after she began taking this drug is strong circumstantial evidence that this drug is likely the source of her auditory hallucinations, exacerbated, no doubt, by her hearing loss and anxiety—two other factors associated with Musical Ear syndrome.

"Joy" was suspicious her auditory hallucinations were connected to the drugs she was taking. She explains:

I have auditory hallucinations that are quite vivid, and I sometimes think I can understand the voices. I have been hard of hearing since childhood and now wear two hearing aids. Lately my hearing has been getting worse.

For the past 7 months I have been changing medications to try to control my blood pressure. In March, my doctors finally found a combination that worked. Since then, the music has become much more profound. **I think the medication is to blame**. I am taking **Metoprolol** (*Toprol*), **Diltiazem** (*Cardizem*) and **Clonidine**. **I believe the Clonidine is the culprit** because it also has caused vivid dreams, nightmares and auditory hallucinations.

"Joy" is very likely correct in her suspicions. Auditory hallucinations occur in a minimum of 5% of the people taking **Clonidine**. The true figure may be much higher. However, **Metoprolol** (*Toprol*) and **Diltiazem** (*Cardizem*) can also cause hallucinations in some people.

"Clara" also wondered if there was a connection between the drugs her mother was taking and her auditory hallucinations. She wrote:

My 76 year old mother has been suffering from auditory hallucinations every waking moment for the past 4 years. She has a 45% to 50% hearing loss in both ears. Extensive psychiatric evaluations all proved negative. She is not schizophrenic, does not suffer from dementia and has no evidence of Alzheimer's. She does not hear voices of anyone talking to her or telling her bad things, merely sentences or songs being replayed over and over again. Although mentally quite sharp, she has practically lost all ability to concentrate. Recently, these hallucinations have been getting worse. These

Key to Drug Names

Throughout this book, the generic names of drugs are capitalized and shown in bold (**Mirtazapine**), while specific brand names are capitalized and shown in italics (*Remeron*).

phantom sounds **began within days of her taking extensive chemotherapy**.

She sleeps with music playing all night long to help drown out the sounds including whooshing, clicking, ringing and air rushing through her head.

She says that *Ambien* (sleep medication) is the only thing that gives her any relief and it's not hard to figure out how that helps. She now takes *Ambien* night and day and stays in a semi-zombie state. In other words, there is no quality of life.

In this lady's case, it appears that chemotherapy was largely responsible for both her hearing loss and the resulting auditory hallucinations. However, the **Zolpidem** (*Ambien*) she now takes may be causing her hallucinations to continue and even get worse.

More Numerous Than Previously Thought

Drugs that can cause auditory hallucinations are much more numerous than previously thought. The truth is, there are a good number of prescription drugs that can cause auditory hallucinations or make existing auditory hallucinations worse.

Also, about 450 drugs can trigger tinnitus.[9] In some cases, the drugs may be triggering tinnitus with specific spectral characteristics. The brain then tries to interpret the resulting "sound" as meaningful signals,[10] often of the musical variety of auditory hallucinations.

As it stands today, there is little definitive information available on exactly which drugs can cause auditory hallucinations. Some drugs can cause psychiatric hallucinations since they do act on the brain. However, there are a number of drugs that cause the non-psychiatric auditory hallucinations—often of the musical variety—that many hard of hearing people experience.

Unfortunately, drug reference books such as the *Physicians' Desk Reference* (PDR) do not distinguish between drugs that produce psychiatric hallucinations as opposed to those that can produce non-psychiatric auditory hallucinations. In fact, there is little mention of hallucinations in drug reference books in the first place. When mention is made, drug reference books often just use the generic term "hallucinations" and almost

[9] Bauman, 2003. p. 42.
[10] Bregman, 2002. p. 2.

never differentiate between the kinds of hallucinations produced—whether auditory, visual, tactile, etc.

For example, the 2003 edition of the PDR lists 171 generic drugs that can cause hallucinations but only lists 6 drugs that specifically cause **auditory** hallucinations, namely **Clonidine** (*Catapres*, *Clorpres*, *Combipres*), **Escitalopram** (*Lexapro*), **Methsuximide** (*Celontin*), **Muromonab CD3** (*Orthoclone OKT3*), **Penicillin** (*Bicillin*) and **Valacyclovir** (*Valtrex*).

This is in spite of the fact that other drug reference books, such as the *British National Formulary* (BNF), list additional drugs as being known to cause auditory hallucinations. The BNF plainly states that tricyclic and related antidepressants can cause auditory hallucinations.[11] These drugs include **Venlafaxine** (bicyclic antidepressant), **Amitriptyline**, **Clomipramine**, **Imipramine** (tricyclic antidepressants) and **Mirtazapine** (tetracyclic antidepressant) to name a few.

See Appendix 2 (page 135) for a list of 28 drugs, herbs and chemicals that are known to cause auditory hallucinations as well as 239 different drugs that can cause "hallucinations" but are not specifically listed as causing "auditory hallucinations."

Researchers are slowly discovering that a good number of the drugs listed only as causing "hallucinations" do, in fact, cause auditory hallucinations. In addition to those listed above, here are some more drugs now known to cause auditory hallucinations, the side effects of which are not yet listed in the PDR. They include **Acetylsalicylic acid** (*Aspirin*), **Carbamazepine** (*Tegretol*), **Clomipramine** (*Anafranil*), **Cyclizine** (*Marzine*), **Imipramine** (*Tofranil*), **Pentoxifylline** (*Trental*), **Propranolol** (*Inderal*), **Triazolam** (*Halcion*) and **Tramadol** (*Ultram*). [12, 13]

Here are some examples. One lady reported hearing musical hallucinations after regularly taking **Aspirin**.[14] Another person reported that taking **Imipramine** (a tricyclic antidepressant) also caused musical hallucinations.[15] In another case, a lady realized that taking **Clomipramine** made her auditory hallucinations louder.[16]

As time goes by, more and more people are reporting experiencing auditory hallucinations from a number of drugs

[11] British National Formulary, 2002. p. 25.

[12] Folmer, 2002. p. 1.

[13] Roberts, 2001. p. 424.

[14] Edell, 1998. p. 1.

[15] Fadirepo, ~2002. p. 17.

[16] Eizenberg, 1987. p. 4.

that are not listed in drug reference books such as the PDR as having this side effect. For example, "Arlene" explains:

I had surgery recently for a hip fracture, and I guess the **Morphine** or whatever started music playing constantly in my left ear. I am profoundly deaf along with a tinnitus problem. At least the music is tasteful, but I wish it would go away. It has been suggested that **Morphine** and *Demerol* can cause this problem.

Both **Morphine** and **Meperidine** (*Demerol*) can cause hallucinations, although neither is listed in the PDR as causing hallucinations of the auditory variety. The same holds true for both **Desipramine** and **Tramadol**. "Miriam" noticed that she got auditory hallucinations from taking **Desipramine**. She writes:

I am on a small amount of **Desipramine** for depression as a larger dose makes **music** in my deaf ear.

In yet another example, a 74 year old man took **Tramadol** and soon after began experiencing auditory hallucinations. In his case, he heard two voices singing songs by Josef Locke, accompanied by an accordion and a banjo. Two days after substituting another drug for the **Tramadol**, his auditory hallucinations stopped.[17]

The following drugs are not even listed as causing hallucinations of any kind—yet obviously they cause auditory hallucinations. The truth is, there are a number of such drugs. For example, "Ruby" writes:

My father has a profound hearing loss that may be getting worse. He was recently placed on **Terazosin**. Since starting the medication he hears "music" even when his hearing aids are out.

Up to now, **Terazosin** has not been listed as causing hallucinations of any kind, although other drugs in the same class (alpha-blockers) are known to cause hallucinations. Thus, it is not at all unreasonable that **Terazosin** would also have this same side effect.

Pentoxifylline is another drug not listed as causing hallucinations, yet it does. For example, a hard of hearing 88 year old woman was prescribed **Pentoxifylline** for tinnitus. Within a few days she began hearing auditory hallucinations— a male voice singing various hymns. His favorite was *Amazing*

---

[17] Keeley, 2000, p. 1.

Grace, but he also often sang *Rock of Ages* and *In the Sweet By and By*.

The auditory hallucinations stopped soon after she stopped taking **Pentoxifylline**. When she began the **Pentoxifylline** again, her auditory hallucinations came back. They once again stopped when she went off the **Pentoxifylline** for the second time.[18]

In yet another example, a 45 year old woman with no apparent hearing loss suffered from moderate depression and anxiety following an overload of work. She began taking **Lormetazepam**, a benzodiazepine available in Europe and Australia. After a few days, the woman noticed musical hallucinations in the form of children's songs. Four months later, her doctor cut her dose of **Lormetazepam** in half. This resulted in her hallucinations changing to resemble classical tinnitus sounds such as bells and sirens. The fact that her hallucinations began when she started taking **Lormetazepam** and changed when her doctor reduced her dose suggests that **Lormetazepam** caused her auditory hallucinations.[19]

As the preceding cases reveal, the proof (or at least a very strong indication) that a given drug causes auditory hallucinations is when, shortly after you start taking a drug, you begin hearing auditory hallucinations; then, when you stop taking that drug, your hallucinations go away, but return when you begin that drug again. Thus, if you recently started taking a drug and began hearing phantom sounds, this drug may well be causing your auditory hallucinations, whether it is listed as causing hallucinations or not.

Discontinuing Drugs May Actually Cause Auditory Hallucinations

Strange as it may seem, just reducing the dose or quitting certain drugs may actually cause auditory hallucinations, even though the person didn't have hallucinations while taking the drug in the first place!

Other drugs may have both effects. They may cause hallucinations in some people while they are taking these drugs, and they may cause hallucinations in some people when

[18] *Amazing Grace*…Pentoxifylline-induced musical hallucinations, 1993. p. 1.

[19] Curtin, 2002. p. 1.

they quit the drug or reduce the dose. Benzodiazepines are one such class of psychotropic drugs that have this characteristic. They have been known to initiate musical hallucinations,[20] or prolong existing hallucinations when people stop taking them. For example, musical hallucinations were reported in a 65-year-old woman whose tinnitus changed to musical hallucinations after she began taking two benzodiazepines—namely **Lorazepam** and **Temazepam**—and then evolved into a rumbling noise when she stopped taking these two drugs. In another case, a 57-year-old man reported musical hallucinations beginning 8 days after he stopped taking **Triazolam**.[21]

Furthermore, people that are on certain neuroleptic drugs in classes such as phenothiazines, thioxanthenes and butyrophenones[22] may find that just reducing the dose of these drugs also results in auditory hallucinations.[23]

In addition to some prescription drugs, recreational substances such as alcohol and nicotine may also cause auditory hallucinations, either during intoxication, or during the withdrawal period.[24] Here is Malisa's experience. She explains:

> I had a very strange experience when I quit smoking. For about a week, I'd wake in the middle of the night and hear voices talking with clear words in the living room. I'd get up to look, and no one was there. Once I got over the addiction's hump, the strangers left. I don't miss the cigarettes but sure miss the company!

3. Negative Emotional Factors

A number of negative emotions can induce auditory hallucinations. Such negative emotions may include anxiety, depression, stress and worry.

Anxiety/Stress/Worry

When you are anxious, stressed or worried, your brain puts your senses into a state of heightened awareness. This is necessary if you are in danger and need this "fight or flight" reflex. However, constant anxiety, stress and worry is not what you want during the course of everyday life. In this state of heightened awareness, you may react without taking the time

Benzodiazepines

As a matter of interest, most benzodiazepines end in either "lam" or "pam." They include such drugs as **Alprazolam, Clonazepam, Diazepam, Flurazepam, Lormetazepam, Midazolam, Quazepam, Temazepam** and **Triazolam** to name some of them.

[20] Fadirepo, ~2002. p. 17.

[21] Curtin, 2002. p. 1.

[22] Stedman's Medical Dictionary, 2000. p. 1209.

[23] Fadirepo, ~2002. p. 22.

[24] Ask the Expert—Auditory Hallucinations, 1999. p.1.

to realize what is really going on. For example, Karen, who is hard of hearing, writes:

> I was working as a contract technical writer. I used to hop on my bike at 6 A.M. and ride to work so I could return early because traffic was much lighter then.
>
> At the time, I was under a great deal of **stress**. I had a Rent Control Board hearing set for 10 A.M. the next morning. I decided to ride to work at 6 as usual, then ride over to the hearing and go back to work afterwards. I set my alarm for 5 and went to sleep. I was using a stereo clock radio at the time, set to its maximum volume.
>
> I usually woke before the radio came on, but this time around, the radio began to play, I hit the "off" button and I got dressed and hopped on my bike.
>
> The streets were totally deserted. I stopped to buy a newspaper, then continued on, signed in at 6 A.M. after looking briefly at the clock. I went upstairs and the floor was completely dark, so I turned on the lights, made some coffee for myself and settled in for work. Only then did I take a close look at my watch. It read 3 A.M! No wonder the streets had been empty!
>
> We sometimes find what we are looking for, so I guess my quick glance at the time clock was merely cursory. I checked my clock when I returned home and found it was set correctly for 5 A.M., so obviously I had hallucinated the radio.

David found himself in a somewhat similar situation. Imagine his stress and anxiety when, as a young, profoundly hard of hearing husband, he was left alone with the baby for the first time while his wife was out of town. No wonder his brain played tricks on him too. David recalls:

> I have a profound hearing loss. When my children were babies, I could hear them cry when I was awake and wearing my hearing aid and not too far away. (My problem wasn't with hearing the baby, it was that with hearing like mine, everything sounds alike. Whenever I heard a noise I'd have to go check and see if it was the baby. We live in a big-city neighborhood, and this kept me jumping.)
>
> When my wife, who has normal hearing, went out of town, I rigged up some baby monitors to flash a light right over my head in bed when the baby cried. Whenever I was awakened by this light, I experienced it as sound. I'd "hear" the sound of my baby crying quite distinctly and loudly, wake up, and only then realize it was the light.
>
> I came awake sure from what I was "hearing" that the baby was right in the bed with me, squalling into my hearing aid. Then, as

consciousness increased, the "sound" became what it actually was, light.

When people are hard of hearing, they are often anxious because they think they are missing something important. In this state of heightened awareness, their brains can play some "funny" tricks on them. Gladys, who is hard of hearing, explained:

I experienced the telephone ringing every time I got in the shower. The second I stepped into the shower I would hear the telephone ringing—very clearly—but it wasn't really ringing. I wrote it off as some kind of **quirky anxiety reflex of being afraid I couldn't hear the phone in the shower.**

In a similar manner, Meghan's brain makes her think her dog is barking when it isn't. She recounts:

I have a profound hearing loss in my left ear and a severe to profound loss in the right ear. I experience tinnitus a few times a day.

Most of the time my tinnitus sounds like sirens, high pitched buzzing or just ringing, but sometimes I hear a dog bark all of a sudden, but my dog is outside and I don't have my hearing aid on, so I know I couldn't really be hearing it. Ever since I got a dog, periodically I hear a single dog bark, even though my dog is asleep or outside and my hearing aid is off. I find this very strange.

Jennifer is hard of hearing. When she is anxious, she sometimes hears the phone or doorbell ringing. She writes:

Recently I have been experiencing the door bell and phone ringing when I don't have the TV on. If the TV is on, I look at the screen and if its not ringing on the TV I know its the real phone or doorbell. **This occurs most particularly when I am nervous, anxiously expecting some one to drop by, or just lonely.**

She realizes what is going on and adds:

My guess is my brain is just playing tricks on me.

You don't have to be hard of hearing in order to experience auditory hallucinations. The truth is that many people begin to hear auditory hallucinations as a result of extreme stress and anxiety.[25] Furthermore, auditory hallucinations don't just occur in adults. Children can also experience them when they are particularly stressed and anxious.

One study reported on the auditory hallucinations of 13 children exhibiting a variety of emotional and behavioral

---

[25] Hearing Voices Network. 2004, p. 1.

difficulties. All were experiencing **high levels of stress and/or anxiety** in their lives. The hallucinations gradually disappeared over the course of therapy. The clinical presentation of the children in this study indicated **an association between hallucinations and high levels of stress and anxiety.**[26]

There is no doubt that periods of stress can trigger auditory hallucinations. Stress can take all kinds of forms. For example, food and water deprivation is a kind of stress that can lead to auditory hallucinations. So can lack of sleep. Being extremely hot or cold, which results in a higher or lower brain temperature than normal, can also induce auditory hallucinations. Apparently even something as simple as holding your breath or hyperventilating can induce auditory hallucinations in some people.[27]

The stress resulting from the death of a spouse is another cause of auditory hallucinations. In fact, some people will hear the voice of a loved one after the loved one's death. This may occur as part of the grieving process. Furthermore, people who have undergone severe traumas, such as rape or sexual abuse, will sometimes hear a variety of voices, usually relating to real persons who were involved in the abuse. This is not a psychotic phenomenon, but usually an aspect of post-traumatic stress disorder."[28]

Psychological stress increases the chances of a person experiencing auditory hallucinations. Such stress can include anything that causes a psychological impact such as anxiety or fear, even if it is unfounded.[29] Patty writes:

> I hear sounds like what I call "the vampires are coming" music—from old movies—an organ would be playing. I also hear many recognizable hymns. I have moderate hearing loss and tinnitus. About 5 years ago, I was under **lots of stress**. In fact, I was a mess. **The phantom music started in the second year of the stress.**

"Mindy" is under a lot of stress from various causes. It's not surprising that all this stress piled on top of each other has caused her to hear auditory hallucinations. She explains:

> I'm really beginning to think I'm going crazy. I hear vague music but I can't find anywhere that it is coming from. I hear the same few songs over and over again. They are *Brahms Lullaby*, *America* and *The Happy Wanderer*. If I put my fingers in my ears, I still hear it. I am 60 years old and this is very frightening.

[26] Mertin, 2004. p. 1.

[27] Fadirepo, ~2002. p. 7-8.

[28] Ask the Expert—Auditory Hallucinations, 1999. p.1.

[29] Fadirepo, ~2002. p. 9.

I don't have a real significant hearing loss, but I'm sure I do have a hearing loss in one ear more than the other. I do find it easier to hear people talking if I am looking at them. I have tinnitus most of the time—a high-pitched sound in my ears that sounds kind of like the screech of locusts or tree-frogs in the trees in the summertime.

I have been hearing this music for about a month now. About a month ago I had surgery. I'm not sure if it started immediately after that or not, but I think it was sometime soon after that. The aftermath of the surgery did turn out to be a very traumatic experience.

In addition, my mother died suddenly 6 months ago, which I am still having a very, very difficult time with. Also, my husband and I were in a frightening, freak automobile accident recently, so yes, I am under a lot of stress.

Another thing is that I haven't been sleeping well for a long time. I usually don't sleep for more than 3 or 4 hours before my arthritis pain wakes me up.

Even marital squabbles can bring on auditory hallucinations. She wrote me later to say:

A couple days ago the [phantom] music stopped and then my husband got mad at me and it started again.

The stress from the death of a husband with the resulting loneliness, depression and quiet environment is a fertile breeding ground for auditory hallucinations. "Eileen" writes:

I have a hearing loss and wear two aids. I wake at night with men singing like a barbershop quartet. Sometimes it is very loud, and I can't get back to sleep. It is such a point of frustration. The music began 3-4 months after the passing of my dear husband.

Dede's mother is in a similar situation. Dede explains:

My mother is 65 years old and has been hearing Christmas carols and a variety of church hymns since November She does not have any hearing loss that we are aware of. She does not hear the music in noise but does hear it at night and when it is quiet. The hymns are clear and understandable. During this time she was **going through a somewhat stressful time** due to my father's poor health.

The good news is that often when you get the stress in your life under control, your auditory hallucinations tend to fade into the background.

Depression

As is the case with tinnitus, auditory hallucinations are more common in people with depression. In fact, musical hallucinations predominantly occur in elderly hard of hearing people who suffer from depression.[30] Researchers report a significant relationship between hearing loss and a mood of depression, anxiety and dissatisfaction among elderly people.[31] Thus, treating both the depression and the hearing loss often allows their auditory hallucinations to fade away.

In one case, a 70 year old woman suffered from acute **depression** and **anxiety**. Her auditory hallucinations took the form of songs from her childhood. As is common in such cases, her hallucinations especially disturbed her at night when she was trying to sleep. Over a period of 4 months, her hallucinations changed from just music to voices singing. Sometimes it was a man singing love songs that she remembered from her childhood in Hungary.

In another case, a 65 year old woman with mild hearing loss suffered **depression** bad enough that she tried to commit suicide. At that time, she began to hear hallucinations in the form of melodies from radio programs. The songs disappeared when her depression lifted, and for 3 years she felt well. Later, when her depression reoccurred, she began hearing the phantom songs again. She experienced musical hallucinations during each of her three episodes of depression.[32]

Depression/anxiety and the occurrence of auditory hallucinations often go together. When people who suffer from these conditions learn what is happening, there is often a big change in their attitudes. This was what happened with Mary's mom. Mary relates:

> My 82-year-old mother's hearing has been getting progressively worse over the years. She has lived alone for 7 years since her husband died. She has been treated for a number of years for **depression** and **anxiety**. About 2 weeks ago she started hearing music. She does not hear voices speaking to her. She has heard *The Star Spangled Banner*, *God Bless America*, a number of Christmas carols, and *Happy Birthday to You*.
>
> My mother is having trouble sleeping because of the music. She suffers during the hours when she should be sleeping. With her

[30] Keeley, 2000. p.1.

[31] Eizenberg, 1987. pp. 3-4.

[32] Eizenberg, 1987. p. 2.

hearing aids out, all she focuses on was the music. She thinks she's going crazy.

I'm visiting with my mother right now and read her what you've written about auditory hallucinations. She was **relieved** to hear that she was not the only one. **Her mood perked up immediately**. I repeated to her the bottom line—that she is **not** crazy.

4. Fatigue (Over-tiredness)

When people get fatigued, their brains sometimes trick them into hearing various auditory hallucinations. For example, Mere told me:

I used to hear noises that sounded like a marching band! It was never a recognizable tune, nor did it have a distinguishable melody—just marching band noise. (I used to play in a marching band for years, so I knew it wasn't any of those tunes.) I heard it most when I was working night shift in a hospital. I was in a children's unit, and they were all sound asleep, so it was **very quiet**, and typically, **I was very tired**.

Sometimes when a person is tired, the auditory hallucinations they hear are just plain strange. Sukeshi writes:

My husband has been experiencing strange auditory hallucinations for the past couple of days. Three times in the last 2 days while I was talking to him, he heard something totally different and out of context in my voice instead of what I actually said. All three times it was the same—an ad jingle with some tune, but he could not recollect it. And I know he heard something very different just from the totally puzzled look on his face. And every time he said "what did you just say" and I repeated what I had said, he said, "no before that."

Sukeshi's husband adds:

I don't think I have a hearing problem. My job is a high stress job and I tend to carry the stress with me always; always keeps bugging me at the back of my mind 24/7. I work long hours; typically 11-13 hrs. I lately have been forgetful, impatient, irritable. I had one recent 36 hour work day that included a 14 hr drive (a couple of days ago); the incidents started happening since that day. I have also had a constant headache since then.

Sukeshi later wrote:

I think you were right about the tiredness causing the auditory hallucinations. My husband did not hear the sounds again. I think the rest over the weekend worked.

"Tasha" also noticed that, in addition to stress, lack of sleep brings on her auditory hallucinations. She writes:

> I haven't been sleeping well for a long time. I usually don't sleep for more than 3 or 4 hours before my arthritis pain wakes me up and I have to take a *Darvocet*. But this morning after my husband left for work at about 5:30 AM, I fell asleep and slept very soundly until he woke me up about 3:30 this afternoon. I just realized that I do not hear the phantom music, which **leads me to think that maybe lack of proper sleep could have something to do with it**.

Being tired and experiencing auditory hallucinations is one thing. However, when a person gets **over-tired**, they may begin to experience weird, loud or scary phantom sounds. For example, Lenora explains:

> Since being overly fatigued due to taking an overnight job in addition to a 9 A.M. - 5 P.M. job my tinnitus has gone from a very mild ringing noise to a severe engine motor noise. This has never happened to me before until I took this overnight job. **It only occurs when I am severely, and I mean severely, overtired.**

> It is a very loud motor engine type noise—a loud rumbling noise — something like a washing machine in my head. I take my hearing aid off, and it's there so I know I am **not** hearing an airplane or something. It was so loud it scared me half to death!

I explained to Lenora that she needed more sleep and these scary sounds would go away. Six days later, Lenora wrote:

> After getting much, much, much needed rest, yes indeed, I am doing so much better. Oh my goodness, what a relief! I will make sure I get my rest from now on!

Laurie's dad had a similar experience. Laurie relates:

> My dad is undergoing a recent sudden hearing loss at 81. He is coping with a lot of noise. One night he awakened to **a roar so loud he thought a car or train had run through the house**.

Carolyn had a similar experience. She wrote:

> One night I woke up **sure there was a train coming right through our house**. Duh! We have no train tracks anywhere near! And it wasn't tornado season either!

I've had similar scary experiences too. Sometimes when I get over-tired, I hear a roaring sound that gets louder and louder until I'd swear a truck or train is about to come bursting through the wall of my house. This is totally frightening unless you know what is really happening.

From those I have talked with, it appears this loud roaring sound only occurs when a person is over-tired. Fortunately, as soon as they fall asleep, it goes away. Thus, good night's sleep solves these scary sounds.

Don't confuse the above auditory hallucinations with the weird things that people may experience from time to time in the half waking/half-sleeping state as they are either falling asleep or are waking up. In this "waking dream" state a person may at times hear a voice or "see things." This is not necessarily abnormal. These are "hypnagogic" and "hypnopompic" hallucinations, respectively.[33] Mike apparently has such episodes. He explains:

> I am a healthy 22 year old male with normal average hearing. Occasionally I hear something like auditory hallucinations. While in bed, fully conscious, I occasionally hear very understandable, 3-5 word phrases. I know they are not real. It sounds as though my own words would sound coming from a different person, as if I am hearing what someone else hears when they talk. It is always random things that make sense, just do not have any context—like 3-5 words out of a long conversation ("Oh, that's so expensive" or "A huge, yummy, scrumptious ham" or "The judge would say no"). The words can come from both sexes and any age source and do not seem to have any relationship to anyone I know or anything I have ever done. This occurs about once a week to once a month and 2-3 times per occurrence. I suspect this might be stress related.
>
> I only hear the sounds when in bed. I thought it was only at night, but I heard it in the morning a few days ago. It occurs when I am very tired but still fully conscious. It may be some sort of waking dream without the visual. This seems to happen a little more frequently when I have late nights studying or whatever. That's why I think it is stress-related. I am not taking any medications or drugs at all.

5. Constant Background Noise

Sometimes certain constant external background sounds become the basis for perceiving speech[36] and hearing music. Examples of these sounds include jet plane noise; road/wind noise when riding in vehicles; fans and other motors; and running water. In addition, the incessant rattle of a train's

Hypnagogic & Hypnopompic States

Hypnagogic is a fancy medical term that denotes a transitional state resembling hypnosis; **preceding** sleep; applied to various hallucinations that may manifest themselves at that time.[34]

Hypnoidal is the fancy term that denotes the occurrence of visions or dreams during the drowsy state **following** sleep.[35]

[33] Ask the Expert—Auditory Hallucinations, 1999. p. 1.

[34] Stedman's Medical Dictionary, 2000. p. 857.

[35] Stedman's Medical Dictionary, 2000. p. 858.

[36] Hoffman, 2003. p. 1.

wheels clickety-clacking down the tracks may eventually also sound like rhythmic, illusory, repetitive phrases.[37]

Sometimes this constant background noise begins to take on a musical quality. Christine tells about her mom:

> My mom is hard of hearing. Recently on a trip to Arizona with my dad she commented to dad when they arrived at their hotel that she really enjoyed the music on the plane. Dad said there was no music on the plane. On the return trip, mom started hearing the music again and told dad to listen. He said, nope, no music. Mom told him to put on his hearing aids. He did. Nope, no music. But mom continued to enjoy it until the plane landed.

A similar thing happened to me when I used to drive my old jalopy with the windows open. I'd have the radio turned up so I could hear the beautiful classical music I like. When I'd turn the radio off, often I would still hear the music for miles and miles. The wind and road noise combined in my brain and took on a musical quality. I knew what was happening, but it was very pleasant, just the same.

Here is how "Danny" expressed a similar experience. He wrote:

> Another oddity is that the tunes increase in volume when I am driving on the expressway. This is very peculiar because **the tunes appear to feed upon the noise of the expressway**.

This is also Martha's experience. She is hard of hearing and wears hearing aids. She explains:

> I have been hearing humming music in my head for over 8 years, and it has gotten progressively worse. The music I hear is the humming of different songs (no words).

> I first started hearing it before I retired, when I was traveling 70 miles each way to work on the Interstate. **I associated it with the noise of the tires on the road** at the time. Then I noticed it was a song in my head, or the humming of one. At that time I would hear more of the song, and not just a particular stanza of it. Back then, 8 years ago, I only heard the humming in the car. Then it got progressively worse until I now hear it almost all of the time.

You do not even have to have a hearing loss to hear such things. One man recalls:

> During WW II, I was a passenger in C-47 (DC-3) military aircraft given mostly to hauling freight and the like in the southwest Pacific area.

[37] Boza, 1999. p. 6.

Flights were long and very noisy. I discovered I could hear music in the noise and used it as a form of entertainment. I found that I had no immediate control over the music, but I could "put in a request" and a few minutes later I would often hear the music "requested." I heard a lot of choral music and popular orchestras. If one were lucky, one might have a lot of mail sacks to bed down on, and the music made a very nice sendoff to dreamland. **I just thought it was a normal response to a very much "overdriven" sensory system trying to deal with the auditory bombardment.**[38]

Another man actually tried to **make** such musical sounds come true. He wrote:

I was on a plane, near the engines at the back, in a very noisy spot. I told myself that I would hear music—not just imagine it, but hear it through my ears. I listened for music very hard. At first I only head a couple of notes; eventually, as I strained to hear what was there, I could hear sustained melodies. With repeated practice, hearing the music became less and less effortful. To make a long story short, my dominant experiences were of marching music and male choirs.[39]

This man is not alone in hearing such things and having normal hearing. Jane writes:

For years I've been "hearing" music of various sorts when I lay in bed waiting to go to sleep—a wide variety, from band and orchestral, to Irish folk music, symphony, opera and so on. My only explanation for it was that **my inner ear was making sense of faint but rhythmic sounds in the room, for example, the fan of the air cleaner**. I am 49. **My hearing is and always has been normal**.

Shirley discovered that her auditory hallucinations also responded to the sounds produced by electric fans. Perhaps her auditory hallucinations are triggered by the low frequency sounds emitted by the fans even though she can't consciously hear them. Her cousin Frank explains:

My cousin, Shirley, (81 years old) has experienced musical auditory hallucinations for about 6 months. She has also had a hearing loss for some 7 or 8 years. During the past 6 months the auditory hallucinations have been practically continuous, but at varying intensities.

Apparently the music she hears can be initiated by her proximity to various electrical appliances! Not only initiated, but even terminated when the appliance is switched off. It appears that the source of the "trigger" is the acoustic noise produced by the fan in each of the appliances, viz. a fan heater, an exhaust fan above hot plates, and a fan in a microwave oven. The hallucinations can be started, then

[38] Jenkins, 2002. p. 1.
[39] Bregman, 2002. p. 2.

stopped, by switching the fan on, and then off. She needs to be situated no more than about 20 feet from the source for the "trigger" to occur.

Her musical auditory hallucinations under these conditions are the same as usual. The illusion of music does not completely disappear when these, or other appliances, are inoperative, but is reduced in volume.

6. "Dental Fillings" & Hearing Aids

You've all heard stories of people who seem to hear radio stations supposedly through their metallic dental fillings, haven't you? Such stories have been around for a long time and are quite common. Here are some stories about metallic fillings supposedly picking up radio stations. Gladys writes:

When I first started having tinnitus in my 20s, **I thought I was picking up some sort of radio signals on my dental bridge!** That was the only context I had for the tones I was experiencing.

Bill relates:

It has been many years since I experienced the same thing. In my case it was right on the heels of getting fillings put in. **I heard what I thought were radio broadcast voices**.

Another person asked:

My mother-in-law keeps hearing music/radio stations and other noises (in both ears). **She seems to have become a "walking antenna" since she had most of her teeth crowned.** Could there be a coincidence?

Although stories like these have been floating around for a long time, I'm beginning to realize that a lot of what people thought was their fillings picking up radio stations is, in reality, them hearing auditory hallucinations.

I think that people **want** to believe they are hearing radio broadcasts through their dental fillings, **because, in their experience, the only alternative would be that they are crazy**. It sounds ever so much better to blame hearing auditory hallucinations on your teeth, than to admit you are "hearing voices" and have people think you are crazy.

With all the stories of people picking up radio stations through their fillings, you'd think it would be a simple matter to verify them, but that is not the case. If fact, it is very difficult to find proof for the dental-filling theory. Ron, a technically savvy, yet hard of hearing, electronics expert wrote:

> I have heard of such things all my life—that people claim they can pick up radio stations through the fillings in their teeth. The theory is that the fillings crystallize and form a radio detector—much like the cats-whisker crystal radios that appeared at the start of the radio era. These radios require no battery or power source. They just have a tuning coil, a crystal, and a headphone. However, the headphone makes sound that a person with good hearing can hear. The analogy breaks down when we consider that the filling in a tooth somehow sends electrical signals directly to the brain that the brain can interpret as sound.

If radio signals were indeed picked up by the metallic filling, the signal would logically be sent up one of the dental nerves to the brain. Since the signal would be coming from a dental nerve, the brain would only interpret it as pain, not as sound. This is just one place where this theory breaks down.

There are other possibilities for how this "radio" sends signals to the brain. Randy theorizes:

> People who are hearing sounds/radios from their teeth may be doing so by way of bone conduction. When the fillings are excited by a strong radio signal their minute vibrations could be passed though the bone to the cochlea, where your hearing picks it up.

If this were true, only a person with good hearing would be able to hear these sounds. The person Randy was referring to has a severe to profound loss so wouldn't hear these faint signals in any case. Thus, another theory bites the dust.

There **is** an easy way to prove whether a person is truly hearing a radio station or is simply experiencing an auditory hallucination. Just give the person claiming to hear such signals a radio and tell him to tune across the band until he finds the station that coincides exactly with what he is hearing at that very instant.

Since this is such a simple way to prove or disprove whether a person can really hear a radio station through their teeth, you have to wonder why there is no authenticated cases on record. I have not been able to find even one proven case. This is not to say that dental fillings cannot cause radio reception, just that it is highly unlikely.

Such stories continue to surface, which indicates that there is something going on—it just isn't what they think it is. For example, here is a story that, although blamed on dental fillings, is obviously due to the person experiencing auditory hallucinations. "Helen," who we first met in Chapter 1, relates:

> I have about a 98% hearing loss in my right ear and about 80% in the left. About a year and a half ago, I started being awakened at night by very loud "radio" voices in my right ear without my hearing aids on. These radio voices generally occur when I'm asleep and are so loud in my deaf ear they wake me up. Sometimes I even jump. It happens every night.
>
> It was rather scary because we live in the country and I thought maybe it was drug dealers with sophisticated communication equipment. Every night I now hear our county deputy on his radio. It's annoying and scary because I can distinguish enough of the conversations to hear phrases such as "armed with a knife" and "body of male discovered." This morning the deputy was singing a little rap song when he received a call. Sometimes I also hear music, which I believe is the road crew passing the house in the early morning hours.
>
> I mentioned this problem to my regular doctor, and he laughed and said he'd never heard of such a thing. I told my audiologist at Beltone and he said "No, you're not crazy. I have a friend with the same problem." **Now we believe it's because of metal fillings in my teeth.**

This is an erroneous assumption because it is obvious "Helen" is hearing auditory hallucinations. First, she is almost deaf so wouldn't hear the supposedly faint signals being generated by the fillings in her teeth. Second, she cannot be hearing the music the road crew are listening to as a) she is deaf, and b) they are **not** transmitting music—they are **receiving** it. Third, if the deputy was singing, and thus transmitting so she could pick it up, his receiver would have been disabled by the push-to-talk switch, so he couldn't have heard the call come in and thus stopped singing.

These three reasons alone prove that "Helen" is totally fooled by her hallucinations. However, she continues:

> I've even heard hunters (who aren't supposed to be hunting here anymore because of increased population and private ownership) on their CBs. Generally, they're being chased by security, from what I can gather. I'm usually so half-asleep that it's more a nuisance than something I want to wake up and listen to, however, **in no way is this**

an hallucination. It's very annoying and interrupts my sleep every night of the year.

Again "Helen" is obviously hearing hallucinations. Hunters aren't out every night of the year—nor are security agents out in the dark catching illegal hunters every night either. The clincher is that she says, "in no way is this an hallucination." The hallmark of an hallucination is that you are so totally fooled that you cannot separate reality from your hallucinations. "Helen" is not hearing radios. She is hearing some of the strange sounds that those with Musical Ear syndrome experience.

Rose also thought she could hear radio broadcasts, although in her case she thought she was hearing marine weather broadcasts. Here is her story.

> I hear radio weather reports! My house overlooks a harbor where boats and ships sometimes anchor. I only hear this when a vessel is anchored—not when the harbor is empty. (I usually check to see if there are any ships **after** I hear the radio.) Although I am profoundly deaf, **even without my aids I can clearly hear a man's voice** saying "Good morning, good morning. This is WNEW," and then words about cloudy, windy and temperature etc. not as clearly. The "report" is repeated over and over and over again! This afternoon, I also briefly heard a woman's voice (no good morning!) with the call letters WINS—both WNEW and WINS are actual radio call letters. This has been going on for several days.
>
> Tonight, at about 2 AM, I was awakened by a continuous high piercing vibrating sound, and the "reports" in the background. Of course, I always check the house to see if I can locate something. **I never play a radio because I can't make out the words**. I rarely watch television, so nothing has been accidentally left on.

There are a number of problems with this story too. First, Rose has a profound hearing loss, yet she says, "**even without my aids I can clearly hear a man's voice.**" This is impossible. Furthermore, even with her hearing aids on she says, "**I never play a radio because I can't make out the words.**" This statement is exactly opposite to her former statement that she "**clearly** hears a man's voice." Finally, notice that what she hears is endlessly repeated. Radio stations do not do this. However, this is one characteristic of auditory hallucinations.

Such stories illustrate that what people **think** is their hearing radio broadcasts is really them experiencing auditory hallucinations.

Beth's story has a new twist. When she started hearing musical hallucinations, she didn't blame them on her dental fillings. She blamed her computer! She writes:

> I found your web site and was so relieved to read about auditory hallucinations. I'm having them. I was diagnosed with a severe strep, ear and sinus infection late last week. My hearing, which is usually normal, was almost completely gone for a couple of days and is now returning gradually. In the meantime, I keep hearing an orchestra playing classical music, **usually the same piece over and over again** but not always. I don't recognize it, but it sounds like a group of cellos playing.
>
> The music is especially noticeable when I am at the computer and I **have even suspected that some part of my equipment is acting as a radio receiver**.

Even though the theory seems plausible, she quickly recognized the major flaw in this argument. She continued:

> Since the music I'm hearing is **so repetitive**, that is most likely not the case.

This is one of the keys to separating reality from auditory hallucinations. If it is endlessly repetitive, you know it can not be a radio or TV station. Thus it has to be an auditory hallucination.

Before we leave this subject, there **is one authenticated** case of a 35 year old Vietnam combat veteran who did indeed hear radio stations—not through his dental fillings—but through a piece of shrapnel actually embedded in his skull and brain.

This man started to complain of depression, headaches, and hearing blurred voices and music. Skull X-rays showed metallic shrapnel in the soft tissues and cranial bones of the left parieto-occipital region. His perception of voices and music were matched with stations in the AM broadcast band, and consistently identified the same station in the 560 KHz range.[40]

Here is another strange phenomenon. Some hard of hearing people swear they can pick up radio stations through their hearing aids. Although hearing radio stations through hearing aids sounds weird, it actually happens with certain hearing aids.

For example, recently when I was speaking at an audiological convention, a few audiologists there told me that certain

---

[40] Boza, 1999. p. 7.

hearing aids made a few years ago had a faulty chip, and under certain conditions these hearing aids truly would pick up radio stations that audiologists could hear when they were testing them.

Sometimes just using a screwdriver to adjust a hearing aid can cause it to act as an antenna. Rick, a hearing aid dispenser once told me:

> I remember having an office close to a radio station in Illinois. When I put a metal screw driver on a hearing aid I could pick up the radio station.

Interestingly enough, some new hearing aids still pick up radio broadcasts. Here is Lois' account of hearing radio broadcasts through her new hearing aids. She writes:

> Recently I was at my daughter's new home and my hearing aids picked up a radio station. I was standing next to the window and their radio/TV dish was right outside the window when this happened. I'm wearing CROS aids. The music thing really surprised me.

Later, Lois wrote:

> The first time I picked up a radio station was in the bedroom of my daughter's home in Wichita, Kansas. The second time I picked up a radio station was in Tulsa, OK in my brother's new home. No matter where I went in his home I picked up the station. It never occurred to me to find that station on the radio. I'm not sure if it is the same station in both situations. If it happens again, I will try to gain more information. My CROS aids are about 6 months old. Incidentally, I traded my CROS aids in for another pair after the first incident, so the second incident happened with a different set of CROS aids—but they are otherwise identical.

If you have one of these hearing aids, you, too, may hear real radio stations. Here's how you can decide if the hearing aid is faulty or if you are just hearing auditory hallucinations. First, check to be sure there are no radios on anywhere near you that your hearing aids could be hearing. If not, then take your hearing aids off. If the "radio" stops, the fault is likely in your hearing aids. However, if you take your hearing aids off and still hear the "radio," you are hearing auditory hallucinations.

7. Brain Abnormalities

In rare cases, auditory hallucinations are the result of pathological medical conditions in the brain itself, such as tumors, diseases, infections such as syphilis and Lyme disease,[41] damage from accidents, etc. Therefore, if you begin hearing auditory hallucinations, it may be wise to have your doctor rule out such neurological problems. He can do this by looking at the results of MRIs, CT scans and EEGs. This is because auditory hallucinations are sometimes associated with EEG and CT abnormalities.[42]

Auditory hallucinations can result from seizures such as temporal lobe epilepsy. They may be triggered by unruptured intracranial aneurysms. They may be associated with dorsal pontine lesions, temporal lobe lesions or other structural brain lesions. Other causes of auditory hallucinations arising from central nervous system sources include intracerebral hemorrhages, neoplasms (tumors), arteriovenous malformations, and rhombencephalitis.[43]

Interestingly enough, one of the first things people think about when they begin hearing auditory hallucinations is either they have developed a dreadful brain condition or they are going crazy. This preys on their minds. For example, Jane, who has normal hearing, writes:

> For years I've been "hearing" music of various sorts when I lay in bed waiting to go to sleep—a wide variety, from band and orchestral, to Irish folk music, symphony, opera and so on.
>
> My only real concern is that this could be a sign of an underlying medical problem of some import—such as a tumor, or brain lesion that is affecting my brain in this way now but could get worse.
>
> I have read on other websites that auditory hallucinations of music in people who have no other major factors, such as hearing loss or schizophrenia, are found to be related in some way to lesions of the brain stem, brain infections, tumors benign or malignant, but there isn't a lot known.

Thus, in order to gain peace of mind, have your doctor rule out these causes. This is what Lenore did for her father-in-law. She writes:

> My dear father-in-law has been hard of hearing for some time. He hears auditory hallucinations. **His MRI, EEG and CT scan were all normal. The geriatric psychiatrist tested him and found no dementia.**

Lesion—What's That?

A lesion is either:
1. a wound or injury,
2. a pathologic change in some tissue, or
3. individual points or patches of a multi-focal disease.[44]

[41] Zimmer, 2004. p. 3.

[42] Thorpe, 1997. p 25s.

[43] Roberts, 2001. p. 424.

[44] Stedman's Medical Dictionary, 2000. p. 987.

When you do this, you can rest easier, knowing that you are just hearing the auditory hallucinations that so many elderly hard of hearing people with Musical Ear syndrome experience.

Brain Injuries

Various brain injuries can result in auditory hallucinations. This was "Katherine's" experience. She writes:

> Twice I had auditory hallucinations and found them unnerving. I had a **head injury** several years ago. The brain injury caused a chemical imbalance in my brain. I take **Ziprasidone** (*Geodon*) for this. The first time I heard phantom sounds, I heard a voice for only a few seconds about 2 months after the injury. Then I heard voices about 5 years afterwards. The voices are people that are close to me like my sister, my daughter and my ex husband. The voices never tell me to do something but usually they say conversational things. It has been almost a year since I experienced hearing voices. The last time it lasted for over 2 weeks.

In another case, a man, who had been hard of hearing for 40 years, began hearing continual musical hallucinations in the form of three or four male singers singing familiar songs with accompanying musical instruments **shortly after a head injury**. The songs usually dated from before the 1970s, when he lost interest in listening to music.[45]

A lady began hearing auditory hallucinations, **likely from a blood clot in her neck/head**. She would hear one or more singers and accompanying music in the form of a piano or band. She also heard things such as wartime planes and sirens, the sound of dogs barking, children crying, indistinguishable sounds similar to the murmuring of a crowd and the sound of her sisters talking to each other.[46]

Occasionally auditory hallucinations can occur due to damage to brainstem structures involved in hearing such as the superior olive.[47]

Unruptured Intracranial Aneurysms

Auditory hallucinations caused by unruptured intracranial aneurysms are quite rare, but they do occur. In one case, doctors discovered that a lady's musical hallucinations were

[45] Griffiths, 2000. p. 2067.

[46] Griffiths, 2000. pp. 2067-8.

[47] Hain, ~2002. p. 2.

associated with seizures originating from an unruptured intracranial aneurysm. They corrected this by surgery.

This woman had been having seizures for 2 years. She began hearing musical hallucinations a year after her seizures started. It all began when she was hospitalized for pneumonia. After she was discharged, she developed constant tinnitus. Later, she began hearing musical hallucinations in both ears. She recognized the tunes but could not control them voluntarily. Her music was seasonal. She heard Christmas music during the month of December. At other times, she heard music such as *Amazing Grace*. She had no history of hearing loss or psychiatric illness.[48]

Brain Lobe Lesions

Experiments with electrical stimulation of the temporal lobe (either side, but mostly on the right) have elicited very clear musical hallucinations.[49] Therefore, it should be no surprise that brain damage to the temporal lobe can also result in a person hearing musical hallucinations.

For example, Dimitri Shostakovich, the soviet composer, who reportedly had a metallic shell fragment embedded in his temporal lobe said, "since the fragment has been there, each time I lean my head to one side, I can hear music—different each time!"[50]

Auditory hallucinations in the temporal lobe may also result from things such as brain neoplasms (tumors). Furthermore, although rare, musical auditory hallucinations may reflect temporal lobe seizures[51] such as temporal lobe epilepsy.[52]

Damage to the frontal lobe can also cause auditory hallucinations. Here is "Gretchen's" story. She writes:

I have been hearing [phantom] music for the last two or three months. The music usually sounds like a marching band. Sometimes I hear different sections of a marching band (tuba, trumpets, etc). I find the music very pleasing. I hear the music more often when I am in my car on the highway. At times I also hear "talking." I don't have hearing loss nor do I have tinnitus.

I get a little upset about it as I research the Internet. Some say that it is a predictor of strokes and seizures. Should I be concerned?

[48] Roberts, 2001. p. 423.

[49] McKay, 2002. p. 1.

[50] Boza, 1999. p. 4.

[51] Hain, ~2002. p. 2.

[52] Ask the Expert—Auditory Hallucinations, 1999. p. 1.

Three weeks later, she wrote:

My neurologist is concerned that hearing the music is a sign of aura related to focal seizures.

Just four days later she had a frontal lobe seizure. She explains:

My research was right. I had what they suspect was a **frontal lobe seizure** on Tuesday. I was taken to the ER and placed on **Carbamazepine** (*Tegretol*) and confined to my house for a period of time.

Dorsal Pontine Lesions

Rarely, unformed or musical hallucinations can occur with dorsal pontine lesions.[53] The dorsal pons is an area of the brain stem that lies between the cortex and the spinal cord, at the back and bottom of the head.

In one case, a 57 year old man had an abscess containing bacterial meningitis in the dorsal pons which caused, among other things, tinnitus, hyperacusis and auditory hallucinations.

This man's hallucinations, which he heard in his right ear, took the form of boys' choirs singing folk songs. Interestingly enough, he only became aware these were really auditory hallucinations after several hours. He thought he was hearing a celebration in the schoolyard adjacent to the hospital.

He was treated with antibiotics and his neurologic symptoms continued to improve. Five weeks after their onset, the musical hallucinations stopped. However, this man was left with hyperacusis and a mild hearing loss.

There are at least ten other published cases of musical hallucinations caused by dorsal pontine lesions. Most of these people also had mild to moderate hearing losses. The hallucinations began between 1 and 14 days after the onset of the pontine lesions. In four people, the hallucinations did not go away, but they did change their character over time. The hallucinations in the other six people disappeared several weeks to several months later.[54]

Neurologic Lyme Disease

Musical auditory hallucinations may be associated with neurologic Lyme disease. One 50-year-old woman explained:

[53] Troost, ~2003. p. 3.
[54] Schielke, 2000. pp. 1-2.

For the last 4 weeks I have heard what sounds like a male choir harmonizing in my head. The voices are faint but definitely alto. It sounds like music played quietly during a Mass or Catholic funeral service. Recently, I have been hearing patriotic music and Christmas music.

I have this 24/7 during waking hours. The only time I cannot hear it is if I turn the TV up loud or if I am on the telephone. **I have late stage neurological Lyme Disease.** MRIs have shown **three lesions on my brain.** I have had a hearing loss since 1985 and have worn a hearing aid since then.[55]

Apparently Lyme disease can trigger such hallucinations by inflaming parts of the brain. Curing the disease sometimes also cures the auditory hallucinations at the same time.[56] For example, two women who had chronic Lyme disease, which included progressive neurologic dysfunction, suddenly began hearing musical hallucinations. Both women had normal hearing.

When these women were given intravenous antibiotics, their musical hallucinations disappeared. In one lady, the hallucinations came back when she stopped taking the antibiotics. Doctors discovered that the difference between these two women was that the antibiotic caused an increase in the CD57 lymphocyte subset in the lady whose auditory hallucinations stopped. Doctors associated the other lady's recurrent hallucinations with persistently low CD57 levels.[57]

Maggie also experienced auditory hallucinations in association with Lyme disease. Here is her story:

70 year old Maggie had been plagued with Lyme disease for close to 10 years. Suddenly she began hearing a melody playing on an organ—very loud, but not deafening. This was a song from her childhood, *When You and I were Young, Maggie.* This song repeated itself for hours. In the months to come, she heard merry-go-round calliopes and *Silent Night.* For a few weeks it was *The Star Spangled Banner.*

The music often began when she lay down for a nap or when she drove her car. In her case, the only way she could make it stop was to play the radio.[58]

When she tried a new antibiotic for her Lyme disease, the songs stopped. The side effects of the medication were too much for her. Since she went off the antibiotic, the hallucinations have returned,

55 Musical Hallucinations, 2000. p. 1.

56 Zimmer, 2004. p. 3.

57 Stricker, 2003, p.1.

58 Zimmer, 2004. p. 1.

but they are now much milder than before—often just a few notes over and over again.[59]

8. Cochlear Implant (CI) Surgery

Many people get tinnitus (or their existing tinnitus becomes much louder) in the weeks between the time of their cochlear implant surgery and when they are hooked up. However, cochlear implant surgery can also result in people hearing auditory hallucinations. Lorene explains:

> I was afraid I was going nuts when I thought I was hearing things in my head after the CI surgery. I remember on the morning after the surgery, I was hearing what sounded like some music from a radio. It was not loud, just soft music playing. Sometimes I would think I heard talking between songs, or it could be commercials. I would hear them a bit more loudly before they went back to the soft-sounding music. I thought I still had residual hearing and that the lady in the next bed had a radio going. Turns out there wasn't ever a radio in the room. I asked my mom if there was that morning. She said no. I didn't tell her why.
>
> Sometimes it sounded like it was coming from a radio. Other times I would hear bagpipes playing. Sometimes I would hear some songs I didn't know play the same tunes over and over. It would change every day. One day it would be a radio, the next day it might be bagpipes, the next could be back to a radio, and so on.
>
> I know it is common to have tinnitus after CI surgery—but no one bothered to say exactly what kinds of sounds they were hearing. I suspect that a lot of people use the term tinnitus when they really are hearing various forms of auditory hallucinations.
>
> After hookup, it didn't go away, but it is not so noticeable. I think it is still there but not as much. It doesn't bother me anymore.

Elaine's experience was a bit different. She described her musical hallucinations after her implant surgery as kind of pleasant:

> It sounded like someone was singing very softly to me. Maybe I died and went to heaven? Since my surgery, I have had a slight case of it in my un-implanted ear.

Sean writes:

> The national anthem was the first thing I heard after my implant surgery while trying to sleep. Also, *God Bless America* comes to me,

---

[59] Zimmer, 2004. p. 3.

especially at night when I lay down to sleep. I also get *Stairway to Heaven*.

In Sheila's case, she didn't notice any auditory hallucinations before she was "turned on." In her case, the auditory hallucinations came later. She recalls:

> After I received my cochlear implant, I heard a radio too. For a couple of weeks after "hook up", I would hear a radio in my implanted ear (my deaf ear) early in the morning before I had gotten up and attached my processor.
>
> I could pick up some words and hear music. There was no radio playing in the house at the time. It was so strange to have it "playing" not only in my deaf ear, but in an implanted ear. Implantation destroys any residual hearing in that ear and removes any possibility of the ear receiving any normal sound. After a while, the "radio" went away. I haven't heard it for about 3 weeks now.

A good number of people hear tinnitus and/or auditory hallucinations before they get their cochlear implants, but find that after they are hooked up, both their tinnitus and their auditory hallucinations greatly diminish or go away completely. This is one of the nice fringe benefits of getting a cochlear implant. Rick wrote:

> Pre-implant I used to hear what sounded like someone running their fingers at random on an organ keyboard. Sometimes it was quite a catchy tune! Since I had the CI surgery a year ago, I have had no tinnitus in that ear except very occasionally a low hum when I am tired.

Dori had a similar experience. She recalls:

> I have not heard a single marching song since I was implanted over 4 years ago, and have only had a tiny bit of tinnitus. What a relief. Before my CI, I was buzzing and marching and ringing all the time!

9.   Hyperacusis

Hyperacusis is an abnormal sensitivity to sounds. Thus, a person with hyperacusis perceives everyday sounds as much too loud—often painfully loud. People can have hyperacusis whether they have normal hearing or are hard of hearing. Incidentally, people with hyperacusis invariably have tinnitus. In addition, some of these people also hear auditory hallucinations. In fact, one article reported, "People with normal hearing, including those who have hyperacusis, can also get musical hallucinations."[60]

A number of people with hyperacusis have wondered if there is some sort of connection between their hyperacusis and their auditory hallucinations? For example, Eric asked a group of people with hyperacusis:

Has anyone's hyperacusis increased to the point where they are hearing voices?

Janice replied:

I hear noises every night. It started after the tinnitus. It's more like auditory hallucinations.

Astrid explained:

One day in the first weeks of my hyperacusis, I was home alone and heard old-fashioned music—trumpets, etc. I immediately thought I had left the radio on, so I ran downstairs to see if it was on—all the while trumpets in my head were playing. The radio was off. At that moment, the music in my head stopped. Maybe it lasted one minute. This auditory hallucination scared me.

JB wrote:

Since getting hyperacusis, I've had occasional auditory hallucinations such as hearing a doorbell or other noise that was not there. These almost always come after I've been exposed to more noise than normal. They can occur in quiet or not-so-quiet environments. The sounds range from the sound of a doorbell or phone ringing (temporary, not sustained ringing like in tinnitus) to the sound of a voice speaking one or more words. Sometimes, these sounds appear to be a repetition of a sound I might have heard earlier in the day. They are temporary and do not recur on a regular basis. It could be many weeks between occurrences. These sounds can cause a lot of worry. They seem to come with hyperacusis and/or tinnitus in some cases.

There is no doubt that auditory hallucinations do occur in some people who have hyperacusis. However, I wonder whether other people have been misdiagnosed as having hyperacusis simply because they hear sounds that those around them can't hear. As a result, their doctors assume they have super-acute hearing—and the first thing that apparently comes to mind is hyperacusis.

For example, recently, I was talking to an elderly lady who was **very** hard of hearing, even with her hearing aids on. Out of

[60] Musical Hallucinations, 2003. p. 2.

the blue, she told me she had hyperacusis and consequently could hear sounds from the neighbor's apartment.

I quickly realized that there were two reasons this just couldn't be true. First, I was talking less than 12 inches from her ear and yet she still couldn't hear me. There is no way she could hear any sounds even 2 feet away without her hearing aids on. She certainly couldn't hear any sounds coming through walls from an adjacent apartment—with, or without, her hearing aids. Second, I almost needed to yell right into her hearing aid in order for her to hear me. If she truly had hyperacusis, she would have jumped back in pain.

Consequently, I do not believe this lady had hyperacusis at all. She was hearing auditory hallucinations. This lady did not exhibit any of the symptoms of hyperacusis, but closely fit the profile for people who have Musical Ear syndrome. I believe that her doctor made a wrong diagnosis because he did not understand the true nature of either hyperacusis or Musical Ear syndrome. I wonder if he assumed that since she was sane, she obviously wasn't hearing phantom voices. Therefore, the voices she was hearing must be real. If she could hear real voices when others couldn't, she must have extraordinarily-sensitive hearing (which is hard to believe in a person with a profound hearing loss). Thus, she must have hyperacusis. This thought process may sound semi-logical, but was totally wrong in this case.

———————

The above are the most common causes of people experiencing non-psychiatric auditory hallucinations. I'm sure there are a number of other conditions that may also trigger auditory hallucinations in some people. Therefore, don't be too surprised if you should experience auditory hallucinations from causes not listed above. If you do, I'd love to hear your story.

Chapter 8

Musical Ear Syndrome and the Health Care Community

I regularly receive emails like the following asking for my help.

Dear Dr. Neil: "My mother is 84 years old and has been slightly hard of hearing for a few years now. Recently she started hearing what sounded like someone singing *Ave Maria* over and over again. **Is there anything that can be done to stop the music?**"

Dear Dr. Neil: "For the last several weeks I've been hearing constant phantom music very clearly. It prevents me from falling asleep. **Is there no way to shut it up?**"

Dear Dr. Neil: "My mother has experienced tinnitus for as long as I can remember. Recently, she began hearing constant tunes in her head—a man singing a classical tune. She is so distressed by this and cannot imagine going on like this. **How can she get some urgent relief as she is very depressed?**"

Dear Dr. Neil: "Thank you for your article and for letting us know that my 80 year old mom is not going crazy! She's been telling us (and everyone who listens) that the 'neighbors' are continuously playing that classical music again. **Is there any cure or anything she can do or take to make this stop?**"

Dear Dr. Neil: "For the past few years I have experienced the unbidden music, identifiable and repetitive (complete with applause!) on a sporadic basis. I really thought I had a neighbor with an endless affection for the *Battle Hymn of the Republic*. **What can be done about it? It is starting to drive me crazy.**"

These are just a few of the many anguished pleas for help I have received. Why are these people writing to me instead of going to their doctors for help? The answer may shock you?

Few Doctors Seem to Take Musical Ear Syndrome Seriously

Few medical doctors and even psychiatrists, who should know better, seem to know much, if anything, about the auditory hallucinations many hard of hearing people experience. Even worse, they do not seem to know what can be done to effectively treat them. The same holds true for audiologists and other health care professionals who work with hard of hearing people. Gail writes:

> My father is 88 and has suffered from tinnitus for years. His hearing is pretty bad. For over a year he has experienced hearing music and voices (sporting events, etc.) at various times of the day. If he plays music he can drown them out. We have seen an ENT as well as a neurologist. They are **sympathetic**, but **have no answers**.

In addition to their ignorance of this condition, it appears many health care professionals do not take this problem seriously. For example, "Helen" told me:

> I mentioned this problem [hearing auditory hallucinations] to my regular doctor and **he laughed and said he'd never heard of such a thing**.

"Sadie's" mom had a similar experience when she went to her doctor. "Sadie" writes:

> My mom is hearing phantom music (mostly classical music and all music that she likes). The GP that she went to about 3 weeks ago **did not take the situation seriously**.

"Rachel" wrote to me totally frustrated and almost in tears:

> My doctor really thinks I'm lying about the music I hear!

When you go to your doctor for help with auditory hallucinations, you don't want him to respond, as did one doctor to a patient with a "sister" condition—Charles Bonnet syndrome, **"You'd better not talk about such silly things!"**[1]

"People suffering from musical hallucinations," one columnist wrote, "are given **little help from the medical community**.

[1] Teunisse, 1996. p. 7.

Doctors don't take it seriously, or put it down to tinnitus—but you don't get the *Battle Hymn of the Republic* from ringing in the ears! **These people seldom get the care and sympathy they should.**[2] I echo his sentiments.

Misdiagnoses Are Common

Another problem is that doctors seem to be too ready to pass off the phantom sounds many hard of hearing people hear as though they were psychiatric problems. It seems they do not truly investigate their patient's symptoms to determine whether they are psychotic or not. For example, "Irma" explains:

My mother started hearing what sounded like someone singing *Ave Maria* over and over again. As you can imagine, most people she told thought she was going crazy—**even her doctor**.

"Julia" relates:

My mother has been suffering from auditory hallucinations for 3 years now. Her sounds are more like choirs singing hymns and are non-stop. **Her doctors seem to pass it off as a psychotic episode or mental problem**.

"Harry" writes:

My wife lost much of her hearing and now she hears the same song being sung over and over in her head. Our ENT wants her to **see a shrink**.

"Katherine " declares:

Twice I had auditory hallucinations and found them unnerving. Mine finally subsided. It has been a year since I had the hallucinations. I am not schizophrenic, but **the doctors treat me as such**.

When "Tyler's" father began hearing phantom music, "Tyler" took him to an ENT. He explains:

The ENT had no knowledge of auditory hallucinations when I asked. **He basically said that it was schizophrenia (I'm not sure how he could tell just by looking in his ear)!**

Can you believe this ENT's response? This lack of careful examination of the person's symptoms shows up in misdiagnosis after misdiagnosis. In one study, the proper diagnosis of Charles Bonnet syndrome had been made only in **one of the 16 patients who consulted a doctor**.[3] Judging by the letters I

[2] Zimmer, 2004. p. 3.

[3] Teunisse, 1996. p. 1.

receive, I see no reason to believe the results are any different when people with Musical Ear syndrome consult their doctors.

Phantom Boarder Syndrome

The training doctors and psychiatrists receive makes it easy for them to have a "psychosis mindset" or a "delusional mindset." Because of this mindset, they frequently come up with a diagnosis of some psychosis or other, and consequently often overlook the more likely-correct diagnosis of Musical Ear syndrome (non-psychiatric auditory hallucinations).

For example, back in 1988, psychiatrists came up with a syndrome to describe some apparently bizarre behavior, which they named Phantom Boarder syndrome. They explain that Phantom Boarder syndrome occurs predominantly in women living alone **without** other evidence of cognitive dysfunction.[4] They defined it as a misidentification syndrome—a false belief that other people were living in one's house. However, they failed to investigate **why** this belief came about in the first place. Here is a classic example.

> An 82 year old woman heard noises on the second floor of her house and believed that a homeless person was living there. She was diagnosed with Phantom Boarder syndrome, a delusional misidentification syndrome that can be the presenting symptom in patients with dementia.

> Three months prior to her visit, she began to hear noises on the second floor of her house. She believed that a homeless person had begun residing upstairs. She heard him come into the house, usually at night, walk up the stairs, and move objects around. She had never actually seen this person, and they had not spoken. On a few occasions, she summoned up enough courage to walk upstairs and found everything as she had left it. She had her locks changed twice and called the police on two occasions; the police thoroughly searched the ground without finding any evidence of the intruder. The patient had a hearing impairment and had purchased a hearing aid without formal audiometric evaluation. The hearing aid was ineffective, and she had stopped using it. **She continued to hear the noises even without the aid.**

> The woman was very distressed about her hallucinations and admitted to feeling depressed and frequently crying herself to sleep.[5]

From the above story, I notice twelve parallels between people who experience Phantom Border syndrome and people

[4] Mikkilineni, 1998. p. 3.

[5] Mikkilineni, 1998. p. 1.

who experience Musical Ear syndrome. The salient factors in this story point, not to a psychiatric illness, but simply to an elderly hard of hearing person experiencing auditory hallucinations, and trying to make sense out of what she is hearing.

1. People diagnosed with Phantom Boarder syndrome have **no evidence of cognitive dysfunction**. In other words, they are normal. They are not crazy or psychotic. In like manner, neither are people with Musical Ear syndrome.

2. People with Phantom Boarder syndrome are generally **hard of hearing**. Thus, they live in a world of semi-silence. People with Musical Ear syndrome are also generally hard of hearing and live in quiet situations.

3. People with Phantom Boarder syndrome hear their "strange" sounds even **without their hearing aids on**. In such conditions they shouldn't be hearing anything except very loud noises. The same is true for the majority of people experiencing Musical Ear syndrome.

4. People with Phantom Boarder syndrome **live alone**. One common result of this is that they live in a quiet environment. Living alone in a quiet environment is also a major factor among those experiencing Musical Ear syndrome.

5. People with Phantom Boarder syndrome are generally **elderly**. The majority of those who experience Musical Ear syndrome are also elderly.

6. People with Phantom Boarder syndrome hear phantom sounds apparently **coming from other rooms in the house**. People with Musical Ear syndrome also hear phantom sounds external to themselves, often seeming to come from another room or even outside the house itself.

7. People with Phantom Boarder syndrome hear such sounds **mostly at night when it is otherwise quiet**. People experiencing Musical Ear syndrome are also much more aware of their phantom sounds at night when it is quiet.

8. People with Phantom Boarder syndrome believe that what they are experiencing is **real** because the sounds appear so vivid and lifelike. This is the definition of a true hallucination. People with Musical Ear syndrome feel the same way.

9. People with Phantom Boarder syndrome **behave in a rational manner** based on their belief that what they are hearing is real. Notice that the lady in the above example changed her locks and called the police. This is rational behavior if you believe someone is intruding into your house. This is the same rational kind of behavior people with Musical Ear syndrome pursue when they hear phantom sounds that are so lifelike they can't tell them from real sounds.

10. People with Phantom Boarder syndrome hear these sounds, not just once, but **for a number of days, weeks or months**. Most people that experience Musical Ear syndrome also hear phantom sounds for days, weeks or months.

11. When people with Phantom Boarder syndrome go to investigate, they find **nothing amiss**. People with Musical Ear syndrome do this too. This is how they eventually realize they are really experiencing auditory hallucinations.

12. People with Phantom Boarder syndrome are distressed and depressed by what they are hearing. Depression is also a common factor in those with Musical Ear syndrome. As you would expect, many people, hearing strange phantom sounds that they cannot put their finger on, become anxious and distressed about these sounds.

It should be obvious by now that the various factors ascribed to Phantom Boarder syndrome just as easily (and, I believe, more correctly) apply to hard of hearing people experiencing Musical Ear syndrome.

I believe the woman in the above example was both misdiagnosed and consequently mistreated. Doctors and health care professionals need to learn about Musical Ear syndrome and rule it out **before** they proceed with a diagnosis of some sort of delusional psychosis.

Too many doctors, when encountering people with Musical Ear syndrome, just seem to shrug them off and don't effectively help their patients because they don't have a clue what the underlying problem is, and don't want to appear ignorant in front of their patients. "Sonya" writes:

> My dad, who is 90, has just recently begun hearing loud opera music
> repeatedly throughout the day and night. It is the same "aria" over

and over. My dad asked the ENT doctor if he had any suggestions or medications because it is very stressful for him to hear the singing. The **doctor told him there was nothing he could do, nor did he explain what the problem might be**."

When health care professionals encounter a person hearing phantom sounds, a common response is to put the patient on some anti-psychotic drugs instead of accurately diagnosing the real problem. "Betsy" explains:

My mother hears music almost constantly at different sound levels. She is in her mid 80's. We are in NYC and **her doctors have never heard of it**. I am quite surprised. One doctor suggested that it might be a **form of dementia**, I'm not sure I believe that. **Her doctor has prescribed the anti-psychotic Zyprexa** and I'm concerned whether she even needs a drug.

"Arlene" wrote:

I had surgery recently for a hip fracture and I guess the **Morphine** or whatever started music playing constantly in my left ear. I love my ENT people but **all they do is offer mind-altering drugs and a pat on the back**.

Putting a sane person on anti-psychotic drugs is ridiculous. It does not cure the underlying problem and may actually cause them to become psychotic. "Tamara" asks:

My mom is 84 and has had a hearing loss for many years. This last year she started hearing music and now voices. Initially she shouted at them to go away but now seems to "engage" them—even yells at me "didn't you hear him—can't you hear him?" These voices seem to describe situations my mom feels need help (hurt kitty in basement, etc). Distractions sometimes help but she's alone during the day, confined to a wheel chair and I feel this exacerbates the problem. Is there some way to help her cope with this so as not to "lose" her to these voices. My mom was put on *Celexa* for anxiety four weeks ago. Could this have any relation to her problem? It does coincide with her hearing "voices."

In this case, "Tamara's" concerns could be well-founded. **Citalopram** (*Celexa*) is a selective serotonin reuptake inhibitor (SSRI) which belongs to a class of psychotropic drugs. Such drugs may affect the mental health of some people while they are taking them. Furthermore, **Citalopram** is known to **cause** hallucinations.

Looking on the Brighter Side

Fortunately, not all doctors hold such caviler attitudes towards people experiencing auditory hallucinations. Some are very concerned and do all they can to help their patients—even when confronted with such strange and baffling cases as Musical Ear syndrome. There are some good doctors, who, even if they don't know what is going on, realize that non-psychiatric auditory hallucinations do not make a person psychotic and take the time to find the answers. Carol explains:

> My Doctor is going to check with his colleagues and let me know what he finds out. **He has no experience of this except in cases of schizophrenia,** but **he assures me that I still have a grip on reality**.

Another doctor took the time to search the internet for answers to help his patient. In the course of his research, he came upon my website. I know this because Kathi writes:

> My 83 year old mother has been severely hard of hearing for the past 10 years. She has been experiencing auditory hallucinations for several years. **Her doctor gave her a copy of an article you had published on this topic.**

My hope is that this book will give many more doctors and health care professionals the tools they need in order to effectively help those experiencing Musical Ear syndrome.

Chapter 9

Alleviate or Eliminate Musical Ear Syndrome

What You Can Do to Help Yourself

You have now learned a lot about Musical Ear syndrome. More importantly, you now know that you are not going crazy. You also know that you are not alone. However, your burning question remains, "What can I do to make my auditory hallucinations go away?"

The good news is that there are a number of things you can do to help bring your auditory hallucinations under control. I've helped a number of people cope with their auditory hallucinations by using the principles laid down in this chapter. As you work through this chapter, you also will likely find that your auditory hallucinations become softer and less intrusive, and may eventually fade away. In any case, now that you understand what auditory hallucinations are, they will make less of an impact on your life.

However, in order to be successful at this, you need to take control and be a part of the solution. Here is what Dede did. She reports:

My mother is 65 years old and has been hearing Christmas carols and a variety of church hymns for the past 2 months. We had all started to think she was "losing it" and thought maybe she needed to see a psychologist until we started searching the web. She has **never** had any history of mental illness, so **we started looking for a reasonable explanation.**

Note

The information in this chapter only applies to people experiencing non-psychiatric auditory hallucinations. If you have schizophrenia or any other mental illness, please seek competent medical attention. Do not try to treat yourself.

The fact that you have read this far shows that you, too, are determined to help yourself, a patient or a loved one.

Don't expect a magic pill to instantly wipe out your auditory hallucinations. Unfortunately, some doctors think that drugs will do the trick. They won't in many cases. Sarah explains:

> My mother is 79 and has been hard of hearing for many years. Recently, she has been hearing the national anthem, and it is driving her nuts. She has been to one doctor who diagnosed it as tinnitus. **He gave her medication and said that it should go away within 3 days. It didn't.** After still hearing the music, so loud that she cannot sleep or concentrate, she went to a second doctor. **The second doctor gave her medication and said that it should go away.**

Finding the solution that works for you may take a bit of effort. Some strategies work for some people and others work for other people. It depends on the exact nature of your auditory hallucinations. Ernestine began trying several strategies to see what would work for her. She writes:

> 1. Yesterday I turned the TV on louder to show the "phantom" that I'm not aurally deprived. So far no change.
>
> 2. Last night I tried to fall asleep with the radio tuned to classic music, but it seemed just as intrusive.
>
> 3. I also tried to make friends with the "phantom" and adopt a sweet, tolerant attitude but after a while I felt like knocking my head against the wall.

Ernestine has the right idea. However, she needs to be patient. Don't expect instant results. Seldom do the auditory hallucinations go away immediately. Persist with the different coping strategies and success will generally come sooner or later.

Following are eight strategies you should investigate as you seek to reduce or eliminate your auditory hallucinations.

1. Seek Competent Medical Attention to Rule Out Brain Disorders & Other Medical Conditions

There is a small chance that you may have a brain tumor or other brain abnormality that is causing your auditory hallucinations. You would do well to have yourself checked out by a neurologist to be sure there are no physical problems in your brain. You may need to have tests like MRIs, CT scans or EEGs to rule out such possibilities.

This is especially important if you do not fit the three main parts of the profile for people with Musical Ear syndrome— namely, you are elderly; you have a significant hearing loss; and you get little sound stimulation because you either live alone or live in a quiet environment.

If you are younger, have normal or near normal hearing and have adequate sound stimulation, yet hear auditory hallucinations, there is a greater chance that some brain condition may be a causative factor.

You also should have a neurologist check you out if you have any conditions that can affect your brain, such as meningitis or Lyme disease or if you were in an accident that caused any brain damage.

At the same time, if you doubt your sanity or grip on reality, by all means, have a psychiatrist check out your mental status. It is possible for a person to have a mental illness **and** hear non-psychiatric auditory hallucinations at the same time.

2. Rule Out Drugs/Change Your Medication

There are many drugs that can cause auditory hallucinations. Appendix 2 lists 28 drugs/herbs/chemicals that are known to cause auditory hallucinations. It also lists another 237 drugs that can cause hallucinations of one kind or another, including auditory hallucinations.

Thus, if you experience auditory hallucinations and take any drugs or medications, you would do well to be suspicious of the drug(s), especially if you began hearing auditory hallucinations shortly after beginning a new medication or changing the dose of an existing one. For example, "Irma" writes:

My mother recently started hearing what sounded like someone singing "Ave Maria" over and over again. **Her doctor reduced some medications and changed her blood pressure medication. The music started shortly thereafter.**

I suggested that one or more of the medications her mother was now taking were causing the musical hallucinations.

Among other drugs, she was taking two medications known to cause hallucinations—**Lansoprazole** and **Metoprolol**. Six weeks later, "Irma" again wrote me:

> I wanted you to know that **my mother's doctor took her off** *Lotrel*, **and subsequently her musical hallucinations went away**. I don't know exactly the time between the two, but I think it was a pretty close connection.

The interesting thing in this case is that although both **Lansoprazole** and **Metoprolol** are both known to cause hallucinations, it appears that it was the *Lotrel* (a combination of **Amlodipine** and **Benazepril**) she was taking that actually caused the auditory hallucinations. Even more interesting is the fact that neither **Amlodipine** or **Benazepril** are listed as causing hallucinations of any kind—although they both can cause tinnitus.

This shows how little is really known about drugs that cause non-psychiatric auditory hallucinations. As a result, if you change any of your medications and shortly thereafter begin experiencing phantom sounds, you should be suspicious of that drug.

In another case, "Pearl" explains:

> I wake at night with men singing like a barbershop quartet. Sometimes it is very loud and I can't get back to sleep. The medications I take are *Cozaar*, **Propranolol**, **Verapamil**, *Lasix*, *Zoloft*, **Amitriptyline**, *Celebrex*, *Prilosec*, **Levoxyl** and *Fioricet*.

"Pearl" is taking 10 medications of which 4 are known to cause hallucinations [**Propranolol**, **Sertraline** (*Zoloft*), **Amitriptyline** and **Omeprazole** (*Prilosec*)]. One or more of these may be the culprits.

At the same time, 9 of these medications can cause tinnitus [**Losartan** (*Cozaar*), **Propranolol**, **Verapamil**, **Furosemide** (*Lasix*), **Sertraline** (*Zoloft*), **Amitriptyline**, **Celecoxib** (*Celebrex*), **Omeprazole** (*Prilosec*) and **Butalbital** (*Fioricet*)]. Since musical hallucinations and tinnitus almost always go together, by taking 9 drugs that can cause tinnitus, 4 of which can also cause hallucinations, "Pearl" could well have set her ears up for hearing all sorts of weird sounds.

The important thing is to **work together with your doctor** to find the best solution that reduces or eliminates your auditory hallucinations and yet addresses the health problems for which you were taking the drugs in the first place.

If any of the drugs you are taking are causing your hallucinations, treating these hallucinations could be very simple. Here are five possibilities.

1. Do nothing. Remain on your current drug regimen and put up with the phantom sounds. You may want to do this if they are pleasant and do not particularly bother you.

2. Stop taking the offending drug—with your doctors permission, of course.

3. Ask your doctor to reduce the dose to a level where it no longer causes hallucinations, if this is possible. Sometimes reducing the dose is all that is necessary.

4. Have your doctor switch your medication to a drug that does not cause you to have auditory hallucinations.

5. If the above are not possible, then you may want to try one of the drugs that are supposed to suppress auditory hallucinations.

Doctors use certain drugs to try to suppress auditory hallucinations—especially in people with Parkinson's disease, whose hallucinations are often caused by the anti-Parkinson drugs they are taking in the first place. Some of the drugs that doctors currently use to suppress auditory hallucinations include **Clozapine** (*Clozaril*), **Quetiapine** (*Seroquel*) and **Olanzapine** (*Zyprexa*). Depending on the person, taken in small amounts, these drugs may promote sleep, suppress vivid dreams or decrease/abolish hallucinations.[1]

"Zachary's" father took *Seroquel*. He wrote how the *Seroquel* changed his dad's musical hallucinations "by making it stay on a note (stuck needle effect)" and "slowed down the sound." However, it did not completely eliminate his auditory hallucinations.

3. Learn About Musical Ear Syndrome

The above two sections included things you need to work through together with your doctor. Once these have been looked after, and if you still have auditory hallucinations, you need to work through this and the following sections. These are things

[1] Hallucinations, 2002. p. 3.

you can do by yourself and/or with the help of your family or friends.

Your first step is to learn all you can about Musical Ear syndrome. Study this book. It tells you just about everything you need to know about non-psychiatric auditory hallucinations.

The reason this step is so important is that when you know what you are facing, it reduces your anxiety so you are better able to cope. Then, often a surprising thing happens, your auditory hallucinations go away on their own—or tend to fade more into the background. This happened to Verna. Margaret recounts her friend's experience:

My friend Verna is 84 years old. She has been hearing phantom music for just 1 week. There are never any words. Some of the melodies she doesn't know, but some she does, like *The Star Spangled Banner* and *Silent Night*. At first, she heard the music in the bathroom and thought it was coming from the room next door, but when she started hearing it in every room, she became aware that it was inside her head.

She's actually a pretty witty person and told me that she no longer stands up when *The Star Spangled Banner* is playing. The last time she heard *The Star Spangled Banner* was good timing since she was already standing up! One day she counted 17 songs and knew 9 of them.

Two weeks later Margaret wrote to me:

Verna is **enormously relieved** after getting your letter. She's very grateful to learn that she's not crazy and probably doesn't have a brain tumor. **Now she feels the music has subsided to some extent and is frequently in the background. Because she isn't worried about it, it no longer really bothers her.**

Even learning a little bit about auditory hallucinations helps. Deena explains:

My mother has begun hearing auditory hallucinations. She did say she tries to keep a radio or TV on as she falls asleep, but the other day she mentioned that the music became louder than the radio. I know **she already feels better and is less depressed after I read your article to her**.

The same thing happened with Karen and her father. She wrote:

I was **so relieved** to find your article which explained what my father has been trying to describe to family, friends and neighbors for several months. He believed the "music" was coming from his neighbor's house.

He is 89 and was a machinist all his life and now has 75% loss in one ear and 25% in the other. and is on 9 medications. We want to rule out the meds (or not) so we can either adjust the meds or leave them alone and enjoy the tunes.

Knowing it is not a sign of mental illness is **such a relief** regardless of the possibility it may be medicine-induced. I know **my father is especially appreciative as he is going to show another retiree and many others, I am sure, in his retirement community your article.**

A bit of knowledge concerning auditory hallucinations also brought Marcy great relief. Marcy writes:

I just wanted to thank you for the piece you wrote on auditory hallucinations. **I was greatly relieved.** I had just come back in from going outside to tell my husband that I was really afraid I was becoming schizoid when I searched the Net and came upon your article. It is absolutely amazing—the similarity not only in the tonal qualities but literally in the songs themselves that I've heard compared to the those examples you mentioned.

Don felt similar relief after reading the same article. He explains:

Just found some good, sound and relieving answers to my, shall we say, "Hymns and the Songs from Back Then." I have had, for the past 3 to 4 months, the most calming and repetitive choruses and wind ensembles, usually led by a bass sax and a baritone playing and singing in a low octave, the older Christian hymns and a few oldies from the forties. Now **I feel much relief and I am able to use your paper as information for my distant family**.

The above examples reveal that the biggest need people have is the need for knowledge about Musical Ear syndrome. Just this one step of explaining about auditory hallucinations can be very reassuring, and bring relief to those hearing these phantom sounds, since they often worry that they are going crazy.[2] When they quit worrying, their auditory hallucinations begin to fade away on their own and don't bother them any more.

4. Reduce Your Anxiety/Stress Level (Don't Worry!)

In the previous section, you learned that often just a basic knowledge about auditory hallucinations is enough to reduce a person's anxiety and worry over the strange sounds they are

---

[2] Thorpe, 1997. p 25s.

hearing. For example, a few days after I had explained about auditory hallucinations to Darlene, she told me:

> For the first time I am **not worrying** about this, and **I am not hearing the music right now either**. I have tried to ignore the sounds before, but it hasn't helped. Now that I'm not afraid I'm going crazy, maybe ignoring it will help.

As you work to bring your stress level down, your auditory hallucinations will tend to fade away on their own. This seemed to be the case with Ed's wife. He wrote:

> My wife lost much of her hearing and now she hears the same song being sung over and over in her head. **The music started a few days before Christmas.** The first song was *Silent Night* sung by a very good choir of mostly men. A day later it was the *Vienna Waltz* over and over again so clear it was like being at a musical production.

One month later Ed wrote:

> Since I wrote you, my wife has all but stopped hearing music in her head. About a week ago, it started to soften in volume and in a few days she would only hear it right before bed, but not loud enough to keep her awake. **Perhaps it was the extra stress of getting ready for Christmas** that brought it on.

When you are uptight, anxious, worried or tired, you may notice that your auditory hallucinations are more annoying and intrusive. This can make you even more stressed and anxious. Here's how it all "works."

The seat of your emotions is the limbic system in your brain. Your limbic system "listens" to all sounds and if you have any emotional attachment (such as fear, anger, anxiety, worry, etc.) to a given sound (such as your auditory hallucinations), your limbic system thinks it must be important. (Why else would you have strong emotions about it?) Thus, it turns up the internal volume on your auditory system. These sounds then become more intrusive so you can't ignore them.

At this point, if you become even more annoyed or anxious towards your phantom sounds, your limbic system "cooperates" and turns the internal volume up even more. This compounds the problem and you become even more anxious and annoyed. Your limbic systems again responds by cranking up the internal volume even more, and this vicious cycle continues.

In order to get rid of your auditory hallucinations, you need to reverse this cycle. Here are two important secrets to getting your auditory hallucinations under control. First, do **not** develop any emotional attachment to your phantom sounds. Do not become upset, annoyed or angry at them. Keep a totally neutral attitude towards them. If you are already upset with your phantom sounds, work towards reducing your emotional attachment to them. Second, act as though your auditory hallucinations aren't even there. Concentrate on other things and thus totally ignore these phantom sounds. (This is not easy to do, I know).

When you do both of these things, your limbic system says to itself, "Master (or mistress) doesn't seem to care about these particular sounds any more. Why ever do I have the volume up so loud?" It then turns down the volume a bit. As you continue to remain neutral towards your auditory hallucinations, your limbic continues to reduce the internal volume and your phantom sounds become less and less intrusive until finally they just fade into the background.

5. Don't Fixate on Your Auditory Hallucinations

If you want your auditory hallucinations to go away, you must not focus on them. If you do focus on these phantom sounds, they will become more and more intrusive. This happened to Carol. She explains:

> I think since **I have become so focused on my hearing and ear problems** that I have **developed a new awareness of the phantom sounds** and, of course, **they are more noticeable** when I hear no outside distracting noises.

Without thinking, some people say, "Ignore your auditory hallucinations." However, you can't accomplish this by being told not to do it. It is impossible for two reasons. First, human nature causes you to focus on the very thing you were told not to focus on. Second, in order to ignore something, you have to bring it into your mind so you can tell yourself to ignore it—and when you do that, you are actually focusing on it, not ignoring it!

A much better way is to **focus on the loves of your life**— concentrate on things you like to do. When you are busily concentrating on something else, you automatically quit focusing on your phantom sounds. At this point, you either don't notice them at all, or they fade into the background and are thus not annoying. This is what Dot finds. She writes:

> **When I am listening to other things and conversing, I don't hear it,** although if I make a conscious effort it is there.

Nor is Dot alone. In another example, a 45 year old woman with no apparent hearing loss suffered from moderate depression and anxiety following an overload of work. She began taking **Lormetazepam.** After a few days the woman noticed musical hallucinations in the form of children's songs. The intensity of these hallucinations decreased when she was concentrating on a task or had a conversation.[3]

What can you do? Keep yourself busy with things you like to do—play a game, talk to someone, or read a book.[4] Have some kind of covering noise/music. For example, you can watch the TV or listen to the radio to cover up your phantom sounds. Some people listen to a personal cassette or CD player or radio as they go about their day's tasks. Find out what works for you.

6. Convince Your Brain of the Falseness of Your Auditory Hallucinations

Since auditory hallucinations appear to be so real, they can easily fool you so you don't know what is real and what is phantom. You need to learn which is which. Then, after you become aware of what is happening, you need to convince your brain that you are on to the tricks it has been playing on you. At this point, you can work to convince your brain to stop it. For example, whenever Gladys got in the shower her phone "rang." She recalled:

> I experienced the telephone ringing every time I got in the shower. Note: this was after a period of hearing loss. The second I stepped into the shower I would hear the telephone ringing—very clearly—but it wasn't really ringing. **I wrote it off as some kind of quirky anxiety reflex of being afraid I couldn't hear the phone in the shower.** It finally went away after a couple of years.

Another hard of hearing person, Fred, had similar experiences. He even came up with two good solutions to separate the real sounds from the phantom ones. He explained:

[3] Curtin, 2002. p. 1.

[4] Musical Hallucinations, 2003. pp. 3-4.

First, I took my cordless phone into the bathroom whenever I showered. The phantom phone stopped ringing.

Second, I taught my dog to alert me whenever the phone rang. Then I encouraged him to hang out in the bathroom when I showered. When the ghost phone rang, he ignored it. So did I. After a while, it stopped ringing.

That was Fred's way of proving to himself what was real and what was phantom. However, what works for one may not work for another. Some people have to do **very** creative things to get rid of their phantom sounds. Tom wrote:

My 87 year old mother in law thought she heard the TV playing even though she could not see any picture. She had **unplugged** it—but she could still "hear" it. So she "fixed" it. She **cut the plug off!**

Experiment a bit and do whatever it takes to convince your brain. In some cases you may be able to put a stop to your phantom sounds.

Randy has a bit of an unorthodox way of separating his auditory hallucinations from real sounds. He explains:

For a while after moving from one part of town where there was always some idiot just outside my window playing loud music at 3 AM. **How I tell if it is real or phantom music is to stuff my pillow around my ears to see if the sound is reduced or cut off. If it isn't, it's the auditory hallucinations.**

Mary Lou's solution is much the same as Randy's. She writes:

I sometimes think I hear kids playing outside. I used to run out and look. **Now I just close my ears with my hands and if I still hear it, I know it's me.**

Here's another creative way to convince your brain of the falseness of your auditory hallucinations. Nancy's neighbor experiences strange auditory hallucinations at times. She recounts:

My neighbor is 71 years old and has lost most of her hearing. She told me at one time that she only had 10% but she can hear with her hearing aids if we talk loud and face her.

She lives alone and hears phantom music often. The problem is that she hears motorcycles outside her home at different times but usually at night. She says she hears men talking and fighting outside her home. They beat on her window and house at times. She said they had gotten on top of her house two nights ago.

She calls the police and myself and another neighbor that tries to look after her, and we can never find anything that would indicate anyone was there. We live in a good neighborhood that has never had these type of problems. We have even spent the night at her home and nothing happened.

She is a smart woman and admits that she could be hallucinating, but when she hears it, it is real to her.

In order to prove to her neighbor that these sounds are not real, they came up with this unique strategy. Nancy continues:

We are setting up a tape recorder in her home tonight so she can **tape the sounds she is hearing**. She wanted to do this so I hope it will ease her mind to find out there are not really motorcycles going around her house.

The above stories should give you some good ideas how you can convince your brain to stop fooling you. Adapt them for your own situation. Use the following five strategies to convince your brain that the sounds it says you are hearing are not real.

1. Have others around you who will tell you if they hear the same things you are hearing. If they can't hear anything, then you know it is a phantom sound.

2. Use a tape recorder and record your phantom sounds. When you play it back, if there is nothing on the tape, you know they were phantom sounds. If your hearing is too poor to hear the recording, get a hearing person to listen for you and tell you if they hear any sounds like the phantom sounds you heard.

3. Have the thing that produces the sound you hear with you. For example, if you often hear a dog barking, have your dog near you. That way you can glance over to where he is laying and see for yourself whether what you are hearing is a phantom bark or not. In like manner, if you phone "rings" when you are in the bathroom, take a cordless phone in with you so you can instantly tell a phantom ring from a real ring.

4. Know what you can and can't hear. For example, without hearing aids, you may know you can't hear music from another house, or even another room in your own house. Thus, you can logically tell your brain that such sounds are impossible for you to hear so they have to be phantom sounds.

5. If you are wearing hearing aids, take them off. If the sounds are just as loud as before, they are phantom sounds. If you are not wearing hearing aids, put your fingers in your ears. If you still hear the sounds just as loud as before, you know they are also phantom sounds.

7. Enrich Your Environment With Real Sounds

Auditory hallucinations thrive when your brain doesn't get adequate auditory stimulation. This often happens if you have a hearing loss and consequently don't hear the everyday environmental sounds that keep your auditory circuits "happy." In addition, if you have a significant hearing loss, you may have trouble hearing people. As a result, you may tend to withdraw from social contact and thus have even less auditory stimulation.

Furthermore, elderly people often experience auditory hallucinations because they tend to live in quiet locations such as retirement homes.

The death of a spouse may compound this quiet environment. Now, in addition to living in a quiet location, you have no one to talk to. With no one to talk to, you may not bother to wear your hearing aids—and thus your world of silence becomes even more profound.

Now, since you don't have other sounds for your brain to listen to, you tend to focus more on your auditory hallucinations. This just makes them even more intrusive. Carol, who has normal hearing, has begun to realize this fact. She finds her auditory hallucinations more intrusive because she lives in a very quiet environment. She explains:

> I think it might be important to mention that I live alone, and always have. I am very quiet. My niece and her family think I am extremely strange since I do not have the radio playing all day and I do not watch television. I do not own a tape deck (except in my car) or CD and only bought the TV for when I have guests. So, my life has been quite circumspect and, for much of it, quite silent. Therefore perhaps I notice these auditory oddities more than other people?

Lenore also is wondering about the effect of silence on her father-in-law's auditory hallucinations. She writes:

> My dear 90 year old father-in-law hears loud music when alone in his apartment, oftentimes in the middle of the night. On occasion, he has

heard the music elsewhere, i.e. when he sleeps at our house, but the volume is much less when he is not at his own home. **We wonder if his living alone in a self-induced solitary confinement may be a contributing factor.**

If you live in a very quiet environment and hear auditory hallucinations, the solution is simple. Surround yourself with sound. The more your brain hears, the less likely it will be to perpetuate musical hallucinations. Therefore, give your brain something to listen to all the time—then it can focus on real sounds and quit producing its own phantom sounds.

One of the best ways to do this is to wear hearing aids. Wearing hearing aids during the day gives your brain real sounds to listen to. Just the environmental and other sounds you begin hearing may be enough to stop your brain from manufacturing auditory hallucinations. In any case, the many sounds you now hear will very likely distract you from concentrating on your auditory hallucinations.

In addition, your hearing aids will help you hear better. As a result, you will likely talk to more people. This additional auditory stimulation may be all you need for your auditory hallucinations to begin to fade away. For example, "Hillary" continuously heard baritone male voices singing traditional Scottish songs. When she got a hearing aid, her auditory hallucinations diminished.[6]

If you don't have hearing aids (or in addition to them), use an assistive listening device such as a PockeTalker ™ or FM system and earphones/ear buds (or use a neckloop or silhouettes if you wear hearing aids with telecoils) so you can hear better.

Cochlear implants also often reduce the intensity of auditory hallucinations for the people that have them. Doug writes:

> My wife is profoundly deaf as a result of a prolonged use of prescription painkillers. She has now a cochlear implant but is plagued by constant auditory hallucinations—**better when the implant is on and worse when she takes it off to sleep.**

Hearing aids let you hear the sounds around you. However, if you live in a quiet environment, you may need to add more sound to your environment. For example, leave a radio/TV/stereo on during the day to give your brain something to listen to. Talk shows are especially good because you have to actively

Treatment Parallels

Treating Musical Ear syndrome is similar to treating Charles Bonnet syndrome in that improving hearing is paramount after adequately educating the person about the disorder, just like improving vision is to CBS patients.[5] See Appendix 1 for some of the amazing parallels between Charles Bonnet Syndrome and Musical Ear syndrome.

[5] Thorpe, 1997. p 25s.

[6] Fadirepo, ~2002. p. 22.

concentrate on what people are saying. When you are concentrating on speech, you are, at the same time, ignoring your auditory hallucinations. The same thing happens when you invite a friend over to chat.

For some people, just a bit of quiet background music may be enough to deter their brains from manufacturing phantom music. However, if you have a significant hearing loss, what sounds like quiet background music to you may, in reality, be blasting everyone else out of the building! In such cases, you **need** to wear your hearing aids when playing such music.

Adding sound to your environment may work well during the day, but it gets a bit tricky at night when you have your hearing aids out and are trying to go to sleep. In the ensuing silence, your auditory hallucinations may come back full force. For example, providing background sounds during the day eliminated "Angela's" auditory hallucinations. Unfortunately they recurred at night when she turned off her radio.[7]

If your hearing loss isn't too severe, you may be able to listen to your bedside clock-radio without disturbing anyone near you while you fall asleep. You can leave it on all night for that matter. If your hearing loss is severe or worse, a possible solution is to try wearing earphones or ear buds so the music won't bother anyone else.

8. Become Socially Active

Many people with Musical Ear syndrome live alone in quiet settings. Often a spouse has died and they now have little social interaction. Coupled with a hearing loss, this means their brains have very little auditory stimulation. In the quiet, they tend to focus more on their auditory hallucinations. This causes them to become even more intrusive.

To counteract this trend, become socially active. Invite a friend over to chat, or go out with someone. Now your brain will have to concentrate on your chatter and hopefully let your auditory hallucinations fade into the background. This often works. Margaret writes about her friend Verna's experience.

> When she is busy or listening to something else or talking with people **she doesn't hear the phantom music.**

[7] Thorpe, 1997. p 25s.

Just having people around you goes a long ways towards keeping your mind from focusing on your auditory hallucinations. At the same time, your brain now has real voices it can focus on. Another benefit of being with other people is that it helps lift the depression and sense of isolation you may be feeling. As your depression lifts, your auditory hallucinations tend to fade away.

If the information in this book has helped set your mind at ease and reduced your anxiety so you can successfully cope with your auditory hallucinations, I have accomplished my goal. I believe that as you put into practice the principles given in this chapter, you will gain control over your auditory hallucinations so they will no longer bother you. This should be your goal. I wish you well in achieving it!

Appendix 1

The Uncanny Parallels Between Charles Bonnet Syndrome (CBS) and Musical Ear Syndrome (MES)

There are a number of amazing parallels between Charles Bonnet syndrome (CBS) and Musical Ear syndrome (MES). Here are 22 of them.

1. CBS is a condition characterized by **visual** hallucinations alongside deteriorating **vision**, usually in **elderly** people.[1]

Likewise, MES is a condition characterized by **auditory** hallucinations alongside deteriorating **hearing**, usually in **elderly** people.

2. CBS involves visual hallucinations that occur in, but are **not** limited to, **visually** impaired elderly people.[2]

Likewise, MES involves auditory hallucinations that occur in, but are **not** limited to, **hard of hearing** elderly people.

3. CBS is not a psychotic condition but occurs in psychologically **normal** people. People with CBS exhibit no evidence of dementia or psychiatric illness.[3]

Likewise, MES is not a psychotic condition but occurs in psychologically **normal** people. People with MES exhibit no evidence of dementia or psychiatric illness.

4. It is important that friends and family understand that CBS is a **normal occurrence** in many visually-impaired people.[4]

[1] Jacob, 2004. p. 1.

[2] Gurwood, 2003. p. 39.

[3] Gurwood, 2003. p. 39.

[4] Roberts, ~2003. p. 1.

129

Likewise, it is important that friends, family and health care professionals understand that MES is a **normal occurrence** in many hard of hearing people.

5. People with CBS may have **simple (unformed) visual hallucinations**—see flashes of light, simple patterns of straight lines, or patterns such as zigzags and circles; or they may have **complex (formed) visual hallucinations**—see individual people, objects,[5] groups of people or children, animals, or panoramic countryside scenes,[6] often in bright colors and dramatic settings.[7]

Likewise people with MES may have **simple (unformed) auditory hallucinations**—hear fuzzy, vague or simple sounds such as humming, buzzing, tapping or ringing, or hear fuzzy or vague speech or music; or they may have **complex (formed) auditory hallucinations**—clearly hear speech, music or singing that, at times, is so clear and vivid they can identify the various voices and musical instruments.

6. CBS is characterized by **visual** hallucinations in people who have a **reasonably sudden change in vision** such as that brought on by macular degeneration.[8]

Likewise, MES is characterized by **auditory** hallucinations in people who often have experienced a **reasonably rapid change in hearing**.

7. CBS may be aggravated by **visual** sensory deprivation.[9]

Likewise, MES may be caused/aggravated by **auditory** sensory deprivation.

8. Most people with CBS suffer from **social isolation**.[10] In fact, both **loneliness and social isolation** are significant predictors of, and risk factors for, CBS.[11] Thus, reducing social isolation by encouraging interpersonal contact helps reduce the occurrence of CBS.

Likewise, most people with MES suffer from **social isolation** as they are cut off from society by their lack of hearing. In fact, a **quiet environment and social isolation** are significant predictors of, and risk factors for, MES. Thus, reducing social isolation by encouraging interpersonal contact helps reduce the occurrence of MES.

9. The most important aspects of managing CBS patients are timely diagnosis, explanation, reassurance and counseling.[12]

[5] Hallucinations, 2002. p. 1.

[6] Jacob, 2004. p. 3.

[7] Jacob, 2004. p. 2.

[8] Roberts, ~2003. p. 1.

[9] Roberts, ~2003. p. 1.

[10] Steen, 1998. p. 2.

[11] Gurwood, 2003. p. 40.

[12] Teunisse, 1996. p. 8.

Most patients experience immeasurable relief when reassured that their condition is not a psychiatric disorder, but rather, is a recognized phenomena[13] that is caused by poor vision and is not related to mental illness.[14] This, alone, may alleviate their **visual** hallucinations.[15]

Likewise, the most important aspects of helping people with MES are timely diagnosis, explanation, reassurance and counseling. Most people with MES experience great relief when reassured that their condition is not a psychiatric disorder, but rather, is a known phenomena that is caused by poor hearing and is not related to mental illness. This, alone, may eliminate or at least reduce the intensity of their **auditory** hallucinations.

10. Vision care professionals should ask all elderly patients with impaired vision if they have experienced visual hallucinations (CBS).[16]

Likewise, health care professionals such as audiologists, ENTs and people working with hard of hearing people should ask all elderly hard of hearing patients if they have experienced auditory hallucinations (MES).

11. **Visual** hallucinations (CBS) may be triggered by a wide variety of stimuli such as conditions of general sensory reduction, fatigue, stress, low levels of illumination or even by bright light.[17] Thus, **increasing the lighting** at home is helpful.[18]

Likewise, **auditory** hallucinations (MES) may be triggered by a wide variety of stimuli such as fatigue, stress, depression and low levels of sound. Thus, **increasing the background sounds** in the home and/or wearing hearing aids is helpful.

12. Reassuring people with CBS and explaining that their visions are benign and harmless and do not signify mental illness is so therapeutic that some vision care experts now recommend that **all** blind people, even those who do not acknowledge the existence of visual hallucinations, should be informed of the possibility of their occurrence and advised that if they do occur, the hallucinations need not be a cause for distress.[19]

Likewise, reassuring people with MES and explaining that their phantom sounds are harmless and do not signify mental illness is so therapeutic that I recommend that hearing care

---

[13] Gurwood, 2003. p. 40.

[14] Jacob, 2004. pp. 3-4.

[15] Rahman, 2004. p. 2.

[16] Gurwood, 2003. p. 40.

[17] Gurwood, 2003. p. 39.

[18] Jacob, 2004. p. 3.

[19] Gurwood, 2003. p. 40.

professionals should inform **all** elderly hard of hearing people of the possibility of their experiencing auditory hallucinations, and advise them that if they do occur, they are not a cause for distress. Many elderly hard of hearing people will be relieved that they no longer have to hide their "shameful secret."

13. CBS hallucinations are always perceived to occur outside the body, and may last from a few seconds to most of the day. They may persist for a few days to many years, changing in frequency and complexity. They have no personal meaning.[20]

Likewise, auditory hallucinations due to MES also always are perceived as originating outside the body, and may last from a few seconds to hours or days. They may persist for a few days to many years, and change in frequency of occurrence and complexity. They have no specific personal meaning.

14. Although not as common, CBS can occur in people with normal vision.[21]

Likewise, although not as common, MES can occur in people with normal hearing.

15. In CBS, the correct diagnosis of this distressing, but not uncommon, condition is of utmost importance considering the serious implications of the alternative diagnoses.[22]

Likewise, in MES, the correct diagnosis is very important considering that the alternative is treating a sane person as mentally ill.

16. Although CBS was described first in 1760, it is still largely unknown by doctors and nurses. In fact, between 1760 and 1989, only 46 cases had been reported, yet in 1989 a single study included 60 people with CBS. Thus, obviously, CBS is much more common than previously thought, and has been grossly under-reported.[23] This is partly because of a lack of knowledge about CBS and partly because people experiencing it don't talk about their problems out of fear of being thought nuts.[24]

Likewise, MES (under all its various names) is still largely unknown by doctors, nurses and audiologists. MES too, is grossly under-reported. This is partly because of a lack of

[20] Jacob, 2004. p. 3.

[21] Jacob, 2004. p. 3.

[22] Jacob, 2004. p. 1.

[23] Teunisse, 1996. p. 2.

[24] Charles Bonnet Syndrome, 2004. p. 2.

knowledge about MES and partly because people experiencing MES don't talk about it out of fear of being thought nuts.

17. It is fairly normal for people who start to see things that are not there (CBS) to worry that there is something wrong with their minds.[25]

Likewise, it is common for people who start to hear phantom sounds (MES) to worry that there is something wrong with their minds.

18. People with CBS frequently do not volunteer the fact that they are experiencing visual hallucinations because they believe doing this will label them as crazy.[26] In fact, many conceal their extraordinary experiences from others.[27] One study revealed that many patients do not even consult a doctor about their visual hallucinations. Thus, the incidence of CBS must be far greater than documented, given the prevalence of visual impairment in this predominantly elderly population.[28] A large number of patients in ophthalmic practice only admit to experiencing hallucinations upon direct questioning. Surprisingly, if asked, the **majority** will admit to having experienced visual hallucinations.[29]

Likewise, people with MES frequently are afraid to volunteer the fact that they hear phantom sounds for fear of being thought crazy. The truth is that many are afraid to even tell their families or their doctors about the auditory hallucinations they hear. Thus, given the prevalence of hearing loss among elderly people, the incidence of MES is far greater than anyone imagines. People with MES generally only admit to hearing auditory hallucinations upon direct questioning and in situations where they believe it is "safe" for them to do so. Surprisingly, when they feel "safe," a high percentage of elderly hard of hearing people will admit to having heard such sounds.

19. Doctors are unfamiliar with CBS as a possible diagnosis. Near misses have been reported in which patients were almost confined to mental health institutions.[30]

Likewise, most doctors and audiologists are unfamiliar with MES as a possible diagnosis. Numbers of people with MES have been labeled and treated as if they were psychotic.

20. CBS is frequently overlooked or misdiagnosed by both ophthalmologists and psychiatrists.[31]

[25] Charles Bonnet Syndrome, 2004. p. 3.

[26] Thorpe, 1997. p 24s.

[27] Teunisse, 1996. p. 8.

[28] Jacob, 2004. p. 4.

[29] Rahman, 2004. p. 2.

[30] Jacob, 2004. p. 4.

[31] Steen, 1998. p. 2.

Likewise, MES is frequently overlooked or misdiagnosed by both ENTs and psychiatrists.

21. An estimated 13% of patients with Macular Degeneration experience CBS.[32] Furthermore, the incidence in low-vision patients in an ophthalmology clinic was 11%.[33] It seems the prevalence of CBS in patients with visual impairments varies from 10% to 15%.[34]

Likewise, I believe that **at least 10%** of elderly people with hearing loss experience MES. For example, when I speak to groups of hard of hearing people, I sometimes ask how many have heard such auditory hallucinations and invariably 10% to 30% of the people present put up their hands.

22. CBS generally is not taken seriously by the medical community. 73% of the people experiencing CBS had not mentioned their extraordinary experiences to their doctors. 25% feared their doctors would not take them seriously or would think they were insane. 12% had experienced their doctors reaction as negative.[35] In fact, CBS is still not listed in *Stedman's Medical Dictionary*, even after being described over 240 years ago.

Likewise, MES generally has not been taken seriously by the medical community. I see no reason to believe that the above figures are any different between those experiencing MES and CBS. People with MES seldom mention their auditory hallucinations to their doctors, and when they do, often their doctors do not take them seriously, or even think they are insane. Although non-psychiatric auditory hallucinations have been around for a long time, *Stedman's Medical Dictionary* does not list anything about MES in any way under any name (psychological, non-psychiatric or musical hallucinations). It only refers to auditory hallucinations as occurring in people with schizophrenia, thus perpetuating the myth that all people hearing auditory hallucinations are mentally ill.

[32] Roberts, ~2003. p. 1.

[33] Thorpe, 1997. p 24s.

[34] Jacob, 2004. p. 3.

[35] Teunisse, 1996. p. 7.

Appendix 2

Drugs That Can Cause Hallucinations—Auditory and Otherwise

Alphabetical order by Brand/Common/ Generic/Scientific Name	Generic/Scientific Name for Brands/ Common Names in Column 1	Type/ Frequency/ Kind of Hallucinations
222 Tablets *	**Acetylsalicylic acid, Codeine**	
Acemetacin **		
Acetyldimethylamine	**Dimethyl acetamide**	Aud. Hal., chemical
Acetylsalicylic acid *		Aud. Hal.[1]
Actifed *	**Pseudoephedrine**	rare
Actimmune	**Interferon gamma-1b**	rare
Actiq	**Fentanyl**	1-2%
Acyclovir	(see **Valacyclovir**)	
Advil Cold & Sinus *	**Pseudoephedrine**	
Alcohol		Aud. Hal.[2]
Alemtuzumab		
Allegra D	**Fexofenadine**	
Alprazolam		rare
Amantadine		1-5%
Ambien	**Zolpidem**	infrequent
AmBisome	**Amphotericin B**	less common

Key to the Table

See page 154 for the key to understanding the entries in this table.

[1] Folmer, 2002. p. 1.

[2] Folmer, 2002. p. 1.

Alphabetical order by Brand/Common/ Generic/Scientific Name	Generic/Scientific Name for Brands/ Common Names in Column 1	Type/ Frequency/ Kind of Hallucinations
Amerge	**Naratriptan**	rare
Amicar	**Aminocaproic acid**	
Aminocaproic acid		
Amitriptyline		
Amphotec	**Amphotericin B**	1-5%
Amphotericin B		1-5%
Anafranil *	**Clomipramine**	occasional
Ancobon	**Flucytosine**	
Anexate *	**Flumazenil**	<1%
APO-go **	**Apo-Morphine**	
Apo-Midazolam *	**Midazolam**	1.8%
Apo-Morphine **		
Apresoline *	**Hydralazine**	
Aricept	**Donepezil**	
Artane	**Trihexyphenidyl**	rare
Arthrotec	**Diclofenac**	rare
ASA *	**Acetylsalicylic acid**	Aud. Hal.[3]
Asparaginase		
Atenolol		
Ativan	**Lorazepam**	1%
Avelox	**Moxifloxacin**	0.05-1%
Axid **	**Tizatidine**	more common in the elderly
Azatadine		
Azulfidine	**Sulfasalazine**	rare
Baclofen *		
Bactrim	**Trimethoprim**	
Benztropine		more common in the elderly
Betaloc *	**Metoprolol**	
Betaseron	**Interferon beta-1b**	
Biaxin	**Clarithromycin**	
Bicillin	**Penicillin**	Aud. Hal.
Bisoprolol		

[3] Folmer, 2002. p. 1.

Alphabetical order by Brand/Common/ Generic/Scientific Name	Generic/Scientific Name for Brands/ Common Names in Column 1	Type/ Frequency/ Kind of Hallucinations
Blocadren	**Timolol**	<1%
Boldo	**Peumus boldus**	Aud. Hal., herb
Bonamine *	**Meclizine**	more common in children
Brethine	**Terbutaline**	<1%
Bromocriptine *		
Buprenex	**Buprenorphine**	infrequent
Buprenorphine		infrequent
Bupropion		frequent
BuSpar *	**Buspirone**	infrequent
Buspirone *		
Busulfan *		
Busulfex *	**Busulfan**	1%
Butorphanol		<1%
Cabergoline		
Campath	**Alemtuzumab**	
Cannabis sativa		Aud. Hal., herb
Carbamazepine *		Aud. Hal.
Carbon bisulfide	**Carbon disulfide**	Aud. Hal., chemical
Carbon disulfide		Aud. Hal., chemical
Cardizem	**Diltiazem**	<1%
Catapres	**Clonidine**	Aud. Hal.
Ceclor	**Cefaclor**	rare
Cefaclor		rare
Cefpodoxime		<1%
Ceftazidime *		<1%
Celexa	**Citalopram**	infrequent
CellCept	**Mycophenolate**	3-10%
Celontin	**Methsuximide**	Aud. Hal.
Cephalexin		
Cesamet *	**Nabilone**	2%
Cetirizine		
Cevimeline		<1%
Chibroxin	**Norfloxacin**	

Alphabetical order by Brand/Common/ Generic/Scientific Name	Generic/Scientific Name for Brands/ Common Names in Column 1	Type/ Frequency/ Kind of Hallucinations
Chlophedianol *		
Chloral hydrate *		rare
Chlorambucil		rare
Chlorpheniramine *		
Chlor-Tripolon decongestant *	**Chlorpheniramine**	
Chlor-Tripolon N. D. *	**Pseudoephedrine**	
Choline magnesium trisalicylate		rare
Cidofovir		
Cimetidine		more common in the elderly
Cipro	**Ciprofloxacin**	<1%
Ciprofloxacin		<1%
Citalopram		infrequent
Clarithromycin		
Claritin Extra *	**Pseudoephedrine**	
Claritin Liberator *	**Pseudoephedrine**	
Claritin-D	**Loratadine**	
Clobazam *		more common in the elderly
Clomipramine *		Aud. Hal.,[4] occasional
Clonazepam		
Clonidine		Aud. Hal.
Clopixol *	**Zuclopenthixol**	3.4%
Clorpres	**Clonidine**	Aud. Hal.
Clozapine		<1%
Clozaril	**Clozapine**	<1%
CoActifed *	**Pseudoephedrine, Tripolidine**	rare
Codeine *		
Codeine Contin *	**Codeine**	transient
Cogentin	**Benztropine**	
Cognex	**Tacrine**	2%

[4] Roberts, 2001. p. 424.

Alphabetical order by Brand/Common/ Generic/Scientific Name	Generic/Scientific Name for Brands/ Common Names in Column 1	Type/ Frequency/ Kind of Hallucinations
Combipres	Clonidine	Aud. Hal.
Combivir *	Zidovudine	
Comtan	Entacapone	4.1%
Copaxone	Glatiramer	infrequent
Coptin *	Trimethoprim	
Corgard	Nadolol	
Corzide	Nadolol	
Cosopt	Timolol	
Co-trimoxazole **		
Cromolyn sodium		less common
Cyclizine		Aud. Hal.
Cyclobenzaprine		<1%
Cylert	Pemoline	
Cyproheptadine		
Cytovene	Ganciclovir	
D.H.E. 45	Dihydroergotamine	
Darvon	Propoxyphene	
Daunorubicin		<5%
DaunoXome	Daunorubicin	<5%
Delavirdine		<2%
Demerol	Meperidine	transient
Demser	Metyrosine	
Depacon	Valproate	
Depakene	Valproic acid	
Depakote	Divalproex	1-5%
Desipramine		
Desyrel *	Trazodone	
Dextromoramide **		
Dextropropoxyphene **		
Diamorphine **		
Diazemuls *	Diazepam	
Diazepam		
Dichloromethane	Methylene chloride	Aud. Hal., chemical
Diclofenac		rare

Alphabetical order by Brand/Common/ Generic/Scientific Name	Generic/Scientific Name for Brands/ Common Names in Column 1	Type/ Frequency/ Kind of Hallucinations
Diconal **	**Dipipanone**	
Didrocal *	**Etidronate**	
Didronel	**Etidronate**	
Diflunisal		<1%
Digitek	**Digoxin**	
Digitoxin **		
Digoxin		
Dihydrocodeine **		
Dihydroergotamine		
Dilantin *	**Phenytoin**	
Dilaudid	**Hydromorphone**	less frequent
Diltiazem		<2%
Dimenhydrinate *		
Dimethyl acetamide		Aud. Hal., chemical
Diphenhydramine *		
Dipipanone **		
Diprivan	**Propofol**	<1%
Disodium pamidronate **		
Ditropan *	**Oxybutynin**	
Divalproex		1-5%
Dixarit	**Clonidine**	Aud. Hal.
Dolobid	**Diflunisal**	<1%
Donepezil		
Doprarm **	**Doxapram**	
Dostinex	**Cabergoline**	
Doxapram **		
Doxazosin ***		Aud. Hal.[5]
Doxepin		infrequent
Dristan *	**Pseudoephedrine**	
Dronabinol		>1%
Duraclon	**Clonidine**	Aud. Hal.
Duragesic	**Fentanyl**	3-10%
Econazole nitrate		Aud. Hal., chemical

[5] Keeley, 2000. p. 1.

Alphabetical order by Brand/Common/ Generic/Scientific Name	Generic/Scientific Name for Brands/ Common Names in Column 1	Type/ Frequency/ Kind of Hallucinations
Ecostatin	**Econazole nitrate**	Aud. Hal., chemical
Efavirenz		<2%
Effexor	**Venlafaxine**	infrequent
Elavil	**Amitriptyline**	
Eldepryl	**Selegiline**	6.1%
Elspar	**Asparaginase**	
Emflex **	**Acemetacin**	
Entacapone		4.1%
Ephedrine *		
Epiject *	**Valproic acid**	
Epival *	**Divalproex**	1-5%
Ergamisol	**Levamisole**	less frequent
Ergonovine *		
Eryc *	**Erythromycin**	isolated reports
Ery-Tab	**Erythromycin**	isolated reports
Erythrocin	**Erythromycin**	isolated reports
Erythromycin		isolated reports
Escitalopram		Aud. Hal.
Eskalith	**Lithium**	
Estazolam		rare
Ethambutol		
Etidronate		
Etodolac		<1%
Etrafon	**Amitriptyline**	
Evoxac	**Cevimeline**	<1%
Exelon	**Rivastigmine**	4%
Famciclovir		infrequent
Famotidine		infrequent; more common in the elderly
Famvir	**Famciclovir**	infrequent
Felbamate		infrequent
Felbatol	**Felbamate**	infrequent
Feldene	**Piroxicam**	<1%

Alphabetical order by Brand/Common/ Generic/Scientific Name	Generic/Scientific Name for Brands/ Common Names in Column 1	Type/ Frequency/ Kind of Hallucinations
Fentanyl		1-10%
Fexofenadine		
Flagyl *	**Metronidazole**	
Flavoxate **		
Flecainide *		<1%
Flexeril	**Cyclobenzaprine**	<1%
Floxin	**Ofloxacin**	<1%
Flucytosine		
Flumadine	**Rimantadine**	<0.3%
Flumazenil *		<1%
Fluoxetine		infrequent
Fluvoxamine		infrequent
Fortaz *	**Ceftazidime**	<1%
Fortovase	**Saquinavir**	<2%
Foscarnet		1-5%
Foscavir	**Foscarnet**	1-5%
Frisium *	**Clobazam**	more common in the elderly
Gabapentin		infrequent
Gabitril	**Tiagabine**	frequent
Gadoversetamide *		<1%
Galantamine		>2%
Ganciclovir		
Gastrocrom	**Cromolyn sodium**	less common
Gatifloxacin		<0.1%
Genoptic	**Gentamicin**	rare
Gentamicin		rare
Glatiramer		infrequent
Halcion	**Triazolam**	<0.5%
Haldol	**Haloperidol**	
Haloperidol		
Hivid	**Zalcitabine**	<1%
Hp-PAC *	**Lansoprazole, Clarithromycin**	<1%

Alphabetical order by Brand/Common/ Generic/Scientific Name	Generic/Scientific Name for Brands/ Common Names in Column 1	Type/ Frequency/ Kind of Hallucinations
Hydralazine *		
Hydrea *	**Hydroxyurea**	
Hydromorph Contin *	**Hydromorphone**	less frequent
Hydromorphone		less frequent
Hydroxyurea		extremely rare
Hyoscyamine		
Ibuprofen		<1%
Ifenec	**Econazole nitrate**	Aud. Hal., chemical
Ifex	**Ifosfamide**	<12%
Ifosfamide		<12%
Imipenem—Cilastatin		
Imipramine *		occasional
Imitrex	**Sumatriptan**	rare
Inderal	**Propranolol**	Aud. Hal.[6]
Inderide	**Propranolol**	Aud. Hal.[7]
Interferon alfa-2a		infrequent
Interferon beta-1b		
Interferon gamma-1b		rare
Intron A *	**Interferon alfa-2b**	very rare
Invirase	**Saquinavir**	<2%
Iohexol *		<0.1%
Ionamin *	**Phentermine**	
Kadian	**Morphine**	<3%
Keflex	**Cephalexin**	
Ketalar **	**Ketamine**	
Ketamine **		
Ketoprofen		rare
Ketorolac		<1%
Klonopin	**Clonazepam**	
Lamictal	**Lamotrigine**	infrequent
Lamotrigine		infrequent
Lanoxicaps	**Digoxin**	
Lanoxin	**Digoxin**	
Lansoprazole		<1%

[6] Roberts, 2001. p. 424.

[7] Roberts, 2001. p. 424.

Alphabetical order by Brand/Common/ Generic/Scientific Name	Generic/Scientific Name for Brands/ Common Names in Column 1	Type/ Frequency/ Kind of Hallucinations
Lariam	**Mefloquine**	less frequent
Leukeran	**Chlorambucil**	rare
Levamisole		less frequent
Levaquin	**Levofloxacin**	<0.3%
Levbid	**Hyoscyamine**	
Levodopa		3.9%
Levofloxacin		<0.3%
Levsin	**Hyoscyamine**	
Levsinex	**Hyoscyamine**	
Lexapro	**Escitalopram**	Aud. Hal.
Limbitrol	**Amitriptyline**	
Lioresal *	**Baclofen**	occasional
Lisuride **		
Lithium		
Lithobid	**Lithium**	
Lodine XL	**Etodolac**	
Lodosyn	**Levodopa**	
Lophophora williamsii		Aud. Hal., herb
Lopresor *	**Metoprolol**	
Loratadine		
Lorazepam		1%, Aud. Hal.[8]
Lormetazepam ***		Aud. Hal.[9]
Losec *	**Omeprazole**	isolated cases
L.S.D.	**Lysergic acid diethylamide**	Aud. Hal.[10]
Luvox	**Fluvoxamine**	infrequent
Lysergic acid diethylamide*		Aud. Hal.[11]
Manerix *	**Moclobemide**	<1%
Marijuana	**Cannabis sativa**	Aud. Hal., herb
Marinol	**Dronabinol**	>1%
Marzine	**Cyclizine**	Aud. Hal.
Matulane	**Procarbazine**	

[8] Curtin, 2002. p. 1.
[9] Curtin, 2002. p. 1.
[10] Folmer, 2002. p. 1.
[11] Folmer, 2002. p. 1.

Alphabetical order by Brand/Common/ Generic/Scientific Name	Generic/Scientific Name for Brands/ Common Names in Column 1	Type/ Frequency/ Kind of Hallucinations
Meclizine *		
Mefenamic acid		rare
Mefloquine		
Memantine ***		3% [placebo 2%]
Mepacrine ***	Quinacrine ***	
Mepergan	Meperidine	
Meperidine		
Meptazinol **		
Meptid **	Mepazinol	
Mercaptamine **		
Meropenem		0.1-1%
Merrem	Meropenem	0.1-1%
Mescal buttons	Lophophora williamsii	Aud. Hal., herb
Mescaline ***	Lophophora williamsii	Aud. Hal.[12]
M-Eslon *	Morphine	occasional
Methadone **		
Methamphetamine ***		Aud. Hal.[13, 14]
Methsuximide		Aud. Hal.
Methylene chloride		Aud. Hal., chemical
Methylphenidate *		
Methysergide *		
Metoclopramide		rare
Metoprolol *		
Metronidazole *		
Metyrosine		
Mexiletine		0.3%
Mexitil	Mexiletine	0.3%
Micofugal	Econazole nitrate	Aud. Hal., chemical
Midazolam *		2.8%
Minipress	Prazosin	<1%
Minizide	Prazosin	rare
Mirapex	Pramipexole	3.1-17%
Mirtazapine		infrequent

[12] Folmer, 2002. p. 1.

[13] Methamphetamine, 2004. p. 2.

[14] Methamphetamine, 2003. p. 1.

Alphabetical order by Brand/Common/Generic/Scientific Name	Generic/Scientific Name for Brands/Common Names in Column 1	Type/Frequency/Kind of Hallucinations
Moclobemide *		<1%
Modafinil		1%
*Monocor ***	**Bisoprolol**	
Morphine		<3%
Motrin	**Ibuprofen**	<1%
Moxifloxacin		0.05-1%
MS Contin	**Morphine**	less frequent
MSIR	**Morphine**	less frequent
Muromonab CD3		Aud. Hal.
Myambutol	**Ethambutol**	
Mycophenolate		3-10%
Mylocel	**Hydroxyurea**	extremely rare
Nabilone *		
Nadolol		
Nalbuphine		<1%
Naltrexone *		<1%
*Namenda ****	**Memantine**	3% [placebo 2%]
Naratriptan		rare
*Nardil ***	**Phenelzine**	
Narkotil	**Methylene chloride**	Aud. Hal., chemical
Naropin	**Ropivacaine**	<1%
Nefazodone		infrequent
Nembutal	**Pentobarbital**	<1%
Neurontin	**Gabapentin**	infrequent
Nipent	**Pentostatin**	<3%
**Nizatidine ** **		more common in the elderly
Norflex	**Orphenadrine**	
Norfloxacin		
Noroxin	**Norfloxacin**	
Norpramin	**Desipramine**	
Norvir	**Ritonavir**	<2%
Nubain	**Nalbuphine**	<1%
Numorphan	**Oxymorphone**	

Alphabetical order by Brand/Common/ Generic/Scientific Name	Generic/Scientific Name for Brands/ Common Names in Column 1	Type/ Frequency/ Kind of Hallucinations
Nytol *	Diphenhydramine	
Octreotide		1-4%
Ofloxacin		<1%
Olanzapine		
Omeprazole		<1%
Omnipaque *	Iohexol	<0.1%
OptiMARK *	Gadoversetamide	<1%
Optimine *	Azatadine	
Oramorph	Morphine	less frequent
Orap *	Pimozide	
Orphenadrine		
Orthoclone OKT3	Muromonab CD3	Aud. Hal.
Orudis	Ketoprofen	rare
Oruvail	Ketoprofen	rare
Oxprenolol *		
Oxybutynin *		
Oxycodone		<1%
OxyContin	Oxycodone	<1%
Oxymorphone		
Palavale	Econazole nitrate	Aud. Hal., chemical
Palfium **	Dextromoramide	
Pamergan **	Pethidine	
Pamprin *	Pyrilamine	
Pantoprazole		<1%
Papaveretum **		
Pargin	Econazole nitrate	Aud. Hal., chemical
Parlodel *	Bromocriptine	
Paroxetine		infrequent
Paxil	Paroxetine	infrequent
Pediazole	Erythromycin	occasional
Pemoline		
Penicillin		Aud. Hal.
Pentacarinat *	Pentamidine	<1%

Alphabetical order by Brand/Common/ Generic/Scientific Name	Generic/Scientific Name for Brands/ Common Names in Column 1	Type/ Frequency/ Kind of Hallucinations
Pentamidine *		<1%
Pentazocine		
Pentobarbital		<1%
Pentostatin		<3%
Pentoxifylline ***		Aud. Hal.[15]
Pepcid	**Famotidine**	infrequent
Pergolide		13.8%
Periactin	**Cyproheptadine**	
Permax	**Pergolide**	13.8%
Pethidine **		
Peumus boldus		Aud. Hal., herb
Peyote	**Lophophora williamsii**	Aud. Hal., herb
Phenelzine *		
Phenergan	**Promethazine**	
Phentermine *		
Phenytoin *		
Pimozide *		
Piperacillin— Tazobactam		<1%
Piroxicam		rare
Pizotifen *		
Ponstel	**Mefenamic acid**	rare
Pramipexole		9-17%
Prazosin		<1%, rare
Prevacid	**Lansoprazole**	<1%
PREVPAC	**Lansoprazole**	<1%
Prilosec	**Omeprazole**	<1%
Primaxin	**Imipenem—Cilastatin**	
Procainamide		<1%
Procanbid	**Procainamide**	occasional
Procarbazine		
Procyclidine **		
Prograf	**Tacrolimus**	3-15%
Prolopa *	**Levodopa**	less frequent

[15] Keeley, 2000. p. 1.

Alphabetical order by Brand/Common/ Generic/Scientific Name	Generic/Scientific Name for Brands/ Common Names in Column 1	Type/ Frequency/ Kind of Hallucinations
Promethazine		
Pronestyl *	**Procainamide**	<1%
Propofol		<1%
Propoxyphene		
Propranolol		Aud. Hal.[16]
ProSom	**Estazolam**	rare
Protonix	**Pantoprazole**	<1%
Protriptyline		
Provigil	**Modafinil**	1%
Prozac	**Fluoxetine**	infrequent
Pseudoephedrine *		
Pyrilamine *		
Quetiapine		infrequent
Quinacrine ***		
Ranitidine		rare; but more common in the elderly
*Rantudil Retard***	**Acemetacin**	
Rapamune *	**Sirolimus**	3-10%
Reglan	**Metoclopramide**	rare
Remeron	**Mirtazapine**	infrequent
Reminyl	**Galantamine**	>2%
Requip	**Ropinirole**	5-17.3%
Rescriptor	**Delavirdine**	<2%
Restoril *	**Temazepam**	<0.5%
ReVia *	**Naltrexone**	<1%
Rhotrimine *	**Trimipramine**	
Rilutek	**Riluzole**	infrequent
Riluzole		infrequent
Rimantadine		<0.3%
Ritalin *	**Methylphenidate**	
Ritonavir		<2%
Rivastigmine		4%
Rofecoxib		<0.1%

[16] Roberts, 2001. p. 424.

Alphabetical order by Brand/Common/ Generic/Scientific Name	Generic/Scientific Name for Brands/ Common Names in Column 1	Type/ Frequency/ Kind of Hallucinations
Roferon-A	**Interferon alfa-2a**	infrequent
Ropinirole		5-10%
Ropivacaine		<1%
Rynatan	**Azatadine**	
Salazopyrin *	**Sulfasalazine**	
Sandomigran *	**Pizotifen**	
Sandostatin LAR	**Octreotide**	1-4%
Sansert *	**Methysergide**	
Saquinavir		<2%
Sarafem	**Fluoxetine**	infrequent
Scopolamine		infrequent
Selegiline		6.1%
Septra	**Trimethoprim**	
Seroquel	**Quetiapine**	infrequent
Sertraline		infrequent
Serzone	**Nefazodone**	infrequent
Sinemet	**Levodopa**	3.9-5.3%
Sinequan	**Doxepin**	infrequent
Sirolimus *		3-10%
Slow-Trasicor *	**Oxprenolol**	
Solaesthin	**Methylene chloride**	Aud. Hal., chemical
Sonata	**Zaleplon**	<1%
Spectazole	**Econazole nitrate**	Aud. Hal., chemical
Stadol NS	**Butorphanol**	<1%
Starnoc *	**Zaleplon**	<1%
Sudafed *	**Pseudoephedrine**	
Sulfadiazine **		
Sulfamethoxazole **		
Sulfasalazine		rare
Sumatriptan		rare
Surmontil	**Trimipramine**	more common in the elderly
Sustiva	**Efavirenz**	<2%
Symmetrel	**Amantadine**	1-5%

Alphabetical order by Brand/Common/ Generic/Scientific Name	Generic/Scientific Name for Brands/ Common Names in Column 1	Type/ Frequency/ Kind of Hallucinations
Tacrine		2%
Tacrolimus		3-15%
Tagamet	**Cimetidine**	
Talacen	**Pentazocine**	
Talwin	**Pentazocine**	infrequent
Tambocor *	**Flecainide**	<1%
Tasmar	**Tolcapone**	8-10%
Tazocin *	**Piperacillin— Tazobactam**	<1%
Tegretol *	**Carbamazepine**	Aud. Hal.
Temazepam *		<0.5%, Aud. Hal.[17]
Tenoretic	**Atenolol**	<1%
Tenormin	**Atenolol**	<1%
Tequin	**Gatifloxacin**	<0.1%
Terazosin ***		Aud. Hal.[18]
Terbutaline		<1%
Tiagabine		frequent
Tiazac	**Diltiazem**	<2%
Timolide	**Timolol**	
Timolol		<1%
Timoptic	**Timolol**	less frequent
Tizanidine **		
Tocainide		2.1-11.2%
Tofranil *	**Imipramine**	occasional
Tolcapone		8-10%
Tonocard	**Tocainide**	2.1-11.2%
Topamax	**Topiramate**	frequent
Topiramate		frequent
Toradol	**Ketorolac**	<1%
Tramadol		<1%, Aud. Hal.[19]
Transderm Scop	**Scopolamine**	infrequent
Transderm-V *	**Scopolamine**	rare
Trasicor *	**Oxprenolol**	
Trazodone *		

[17] Curtin, 2002. p. 1.

[18] I have an anecdotal report in my files of a man that began to hear "music" when he was put on **Terazosin** although the PDR does not list hallucinations as a side effect for this drug. However, the PDR does list **Prazosin**, a drug in the same class, as causing hallucinations in less than 1% of the people taking it so it is not unreasonable that **Terazosin** could have this same side effect.

[19] Keeley, 2000. p. 1.

Alphabetical order by Brand/Common/ Generic/Scientific Name	Generic/Scientific Name for Brands/ Common Names in Column 1	Type/ Frequency/ Kind of Hallucinations
Trental***	**Pentoxifylline**	Aud. Hal.[20]
Tretinoin		6%
Triavil *	**Amitriptyline**	
Triazolam		Aud. Hal.[21]
Trihexyphenidyl		rare
Trilisate	**Choline magnesium trisalicylate**	rare
Trimethoprim		
Trimipramine		
Trinalin *	**Azatadine**	
Tripolidine *		
Trovafloxacin		<1%
Trovan	**Trovafloxacin**	<1%
Ulone *	**Chlophedianol**	
Ultracet	**Tramadol**	<1%, Aud. Hal.[22]
Ultradol *	**Etodolac**	<1%
Ultram	**Tramadol**	<1%, Aud. Hal.[23]
Urispas **	**Flavoxate**	
Valacyclovir (Acyclovir)		Aud. Hal.
Valcyte	**Valganciclovir**	<5%
Valganciclovir		<5%
Valium	**Diazepam**	
Valproate		
Valproic acid		
Valtrex	**Valacyclovir**	Aud. Hal.
Vantin	**Cefpodoxime**	<1%
Veetids	**Penicillin**	Aud. Hal.
Venlafaxine		infrequent
Versed	**Midazolam**	<1%
Vesanoid	**Tretinoin**	6%
Vioxx	**Rofecoxib**	<0.1%
Vistide	**Cidofovir**	
Vivactil	**Protriptyline**	

[20] Keeley, 2000. p. 1.
[21] Roberts, 2001. p. 424.
[22] Keeley, 2000. p. 1.
[23] Keeley, 2000. p. 1.

Alphabetical order by Brand/Common/ Generic/Scientific Name	Generic/Scientific Name for Brands/ Common Names in Column 1	Type/ Frequency/ Kind of Hallucinations
Wellbutrin	**Bupropion**	frequent
Xanax	**Alprazolam**	rare
Zalcitabine		<1%
Zaleplon		<1%
Zanaflex **	**Tizanidine**	
Zantac	**Ranitidine**	rare
Zebeta	**Bisoprolol**	
Ziac	**Bisoprolol**	
Zidovudine *		
Zimovane **	**Zopiclone**	
Zoledronic acid		
Zolmitriptan		rare
Zoloft	**Sertraline**	infrequent
Zolpidem		infrequent
Zometa	**Zoledronic acid**	
Zomig	**Zolmitriptan**	rare
Zopiclone **	**Zopiclone**	
Zosyn	**Piperacillin— Tazobactam**	<1%
Zovirax	**Valacyclovir**	Aud. Hal.
Zuclopenthixol *		3.4%
Zyban	**Bupropion**	
Zyprexa	**Olanzapine**	
Zyrtec	**Cetirizine**	

Key to Appendix 2

Typeface:

Bold: Ototoxic drug generic name or chemical or herb scientific name

Italic—Drug or chemical brand name

Normal—Common name of herb or alternate chemical name

Column 1:

No asterisk—information taken from the 2002 *PDR Companion Guide*.

One Single asterisk (*)—information taken from the 2003 *Compendium of Pharmaceuticals and Specialties* (CPS).

Double asterisk (**)—information taken from the 2002 *British National Formulary* (BNF).

Triple asterisk (***)—information taken from other sources.

Column 3:

Aud. Hal.—This abbreviation, if present, specifically indicates that this substance can cause auditory hallucinations. Otherwise, this substance is known to cause hallucinations, but not specifically auditory hallucinations.

If "chemical" or "herb" is not specifically stated, then this substance is a drug.

If left blank or no incidence figures given, then the frequency of occurrence is unknown—just that it does occur in some people.

Literature Cited

Amazing Grace...Pentoxifylline-induced Musical Hallucinations. 1993. In: Neurology 1993; 43:1621. CSM West Midlands re: Action August 1994, No. 5. http://www.csmwm.org/reaction/No5.htm.

Ask the Expert—Auditory Hallucinations. 1999. http://www.mhsource.com/expert/exp1041999f.html.

Bauman, Neil G. 2002. *When Your Ears Ring! Cope With Your Tinnitus—Here's How*. GuidePost Publications. 49 Piston Court, Stewartstown, PA 17363. http://www.hearinglosshelp.com.

Bauman, Neil G. 2003. *Ototoxic Drugs Exposed*. GuidePost Publications. 49 Piston Court, Stewartstown, PA 17363. http://www.hearinglosshelp.com.

Boza, Ramon. 1999. Hallucinations and Illusions of Non-Psychiatric Aetiologies. University of Miami. Priory Lodge Education Ltd. http:/www.priory.com/halluc.htm.

Bregman, Al. 2002. Emeritus Professor of Psychology. McGill University. Montreal, Quebec. Email on musical hallucinations. August 7, 2002.

British National Formulary (BNF 44). September 2002. Published by the British Medical Association and the Royal Pharmaceutical Society of Great Britain. Pharmaceutical Press, PO Box 151, Wallingford, Oxon, OX10 8QU, UK. http://www.pharmpress.com.

Charles Bonnet Syndrome. 2004. Royal National Institute for the Blind. http://www.rnib.org.uk/xpedio/groups/public/documents/PublicWebsite/public_rnib003641.hcsp.

Cohen, Mark & M. F. Green. 1995. Where the Voices Come From: Imaging of Schizophrenic Auditory Hallucinations. Presented at the Society for Neuroscience, 1995. http://airto.loni-ucla.edu/BMCweb/BMC_BIOS/MarkCohen/abstracts/schizo.html.

Cole, M. G., et al. 2002. The Prevalence and Phenomenology of Auditory Hallucinations Among Elderly Subjects Attending an Audiology Clinic. Dept. of Psychiatry, St-Mary's Hospital. Montreal, P.Q. Canada. Int. J. Geriatr. Psychiatry. 2002 May;17(5):444-452. http://www.ncbi.nlm.nih.gov/entrez/query.fcgi?cmd=Retrieve&db=PubMed&list_uids=11994933&dopt=Abstract.

Compendium of Pharmaceuticals and Specialties. 2003. Canadian Pharmacists Association, 1785 Alta Vista Drive, Ottawa Ontario, Canada K1G 3Y6.

Curtin, Francois. 2002. Musical Hallucinations During a Treatment with Benzodiazepines. Canadian Psychiatric Association. http://www.cpa-apc.org/Publications/Archives/CJP/2002/october/lettersMusical.asp.

Deutsch, Diana. 2002. Professor of Psychology. University of California, San Diego. Email on musical hallucinations August 7, 2002.

Edell, Dean. 1998. Musical Hallucinations. December 30 1998. Health Central. http://www.healthcentral.com/drdean/deanfulltexttopics.cfm?ID=8329&storytype=DeanTopics.

Eizenberg, D., et. al. 1987. Musical Hallucinations, Depression and Old Age. Psychopathology. 20:220-223. http://psych.co.il/homeEnglish/2.htm.

Fadirepo, Rinde. ~2002. Auditory Hallucinations. Macalester College, Department of Psychology. St. Paul. MN. http://www.macalester.edu/~psych/whathap/UBNRP/Audition/site/rin.html.

Folmer, Robert. 2002. Walking Antenna, Metallic Fillings and Lucille Ball. Audiology Online. http://www.audiologyonline.com/askexpert/display_question.asp?id=98.

Griffiths, T. D. 2000. Musical Hallucinosis in Acquired Deafness. Oxford University Press. In: *Brain* (2000), 123, 2065-2076. http://www.staff.ncl.ac.uk/t.d.griffiths/music_hal.pdf.

Gurwood, Andrew. 2003. Charles Bonnet Syndrome—Visual Hallucinations in the Elderly. http://www.optometry.co.uk/articles/20031114/gurwood20031114.pdf.

Haahr, Marit. August, 2004. Hearing. The Infinite Mind. Broadcast on August 25, 2004. http://www.lcmedia.com/mind337.htm.

Hain, Timothy. ~2002. Central Hearing Loss. http://www.tchain.com/otoneurology/disorders/hearing/cent_hearing.html.

Hallucinations. 2002. National Parkinson Foundation. http://www.parkinson.org/hallucin.htm.

Hearing Voices Network. 2004. Welcome. http://www.hearing-voices.org.

Hoffman, Ralph. 2003. Auditory Hallucinations: What's It Like Hearing Voices? http://www.healthyplace.com/communities/Thought_Disorders/schizo/articles/hearing_voices.asp.

Holland, Julie, and Kevin Riley. ~2001. Characterizing Auditory Hallucinations: An Aid in the Differential Diagnosis of Malingering. http://www.inch.com/~holland/Julie/papers/paper1.html.

Jacob, Anu. 2004. Charles Bonnet Syndrome—Elderly People and Visual Hallucinations. http://bmj.bmjjournals.com/cgi/content/full/328/7455/1552.

Jenkins, Jim. 2002. Jim Jenkins: Auditory Hallucinations. http://www.auditory.org/mhonarc/2002/msg00296.html.

Juan, Stephen. May, 2002. Phantom Limb Syndrome. In: *Odd News*. Harpercollins. http://www.harpercollins.com.au/drstephenjuan/news_0205.htm.

Keeley, Paul, et. al. Dec. 23, 2000. Hear My Song: Auditory Hallucinations with Tramadol Hydrochloride. British Medical Journal. http://articles.findarticles.com/p/articles/mi_m0999/is_7276_321/ai_69057220.

Lindsay. 2003. Classical Music. http://experts.about.com/q/2272/3324192.htm.

Lockwood, Alan H. 2001. Eye Movements Linked to Tinnitus; Ringing in Ears. American Academy of Neurology. http://www.newswise.com/articles/2001/2/NEURLOGY.VAR.html.

Long, Phillip W. 2003. Chapter 3. Psychotic Symptoms. Internet Mental Health. http://www.mentalhealth.com/books/scz/scz2-03.html.

McKay, Colette. 2002. Re: Musical Hallucinations. http://www.auditory.org/postings/2002/298.html.

Mertin, Peter & Steve Hartwig. 2004. Auditory Hallucinations in Nonpsychotic Children: Diagnostic Considerations. Child and Adolescent Mental Health. Volume 9 Issue 1 Page 9. Feb. 2004. http://www.blackwell-synergy.com/links/doi/10.1046/j.1475-357X.2003.00070.x/abs.

Methamphetamine. 2003. Office of National Drug Control Policy. Drug Policy Information Clearinghouse: Fact Sheet. http://www.whitehousedrugpolicy.gov/publications/factsht/methamph.

Methamphetamine. 2004. Alcohol Drug Association New Zealand. http://www.adanz.org.nz/index.cfm/drugmeth.

Mikkilineni, Sowmya, et al. 1998. Case Report: Phantom Boarder Syndrome. Annals of Long-Term Care 1998; 6(12):401-405. http://www.mmhc.com/engine.pl?station=mmhc&template=altcfull.html&id=1654.

Musical Hallucinations. 2000. The Neurology and Neurosurgery Forum. The Cleveland Clinic. http://www.medhelp.org/forums/neuro/messages/30750a.html.

Musical Hallucinations. 2003. Fact Sheet. Royal National Institute for the Deaf. http://www.rnid.org.uk/html/factsheets/tin_musical_hallucinations.htm.

Musical Hallucinations Linked to Brain Disorders. 2000. Neurology Forum. http://www.neurologychannel.com/NeurologyWorld/musical.shtml.

Physicians' Desk Reference. 57th Edition. 2003. Thompson PDR. Montvale, NJ 07645-1742.

Physicians' Desk Reference Companion Guide. 56th Edition. 2002. Thompson Medical Economics. Montvale, NJ 07645-1742.

Rahman, Imran. 2004. Charles Bonnet Syndrome—Elderly People and Visual Hallucinations. http://bmj.bmjjournals.com/cgi/eletters/328/7455/1552.

Rare Hallucinations Make Music in the Mind. 2000. Science Daily. http://www.sciencedaily.com/releases/2000/08/000809065249.htm.

RNID Discussion Forum. 2004. http://www.rnid.org.uk/ubb/Forum1/HTML/002553.html.

Roberts, Dan. ~2003. Charles Bonnet Syndrome (CBS). http://www.mdsupport.org/library/chbonnet.html.

Roberts, Daniel, et al. 2001. Musical Hallucinations Associated with Seizures Originating from an Intracranial Aneurysm. Mayo Clin. Proc. 2001;76:423-426. Mayo Clinic. Scottsdale, AZ.

Scans Uncover "Music of the Mind." 2000. BBC News. August 7, 2000. http://news.bbc.co.uk/1/hi/health/870054.stm.

Schielke, Eva, et. all. 2000. Musical Hallucinations with Dorsal Pontine Lesions. Neurology 2000; 55:454-455.

Stedman's Medical Dictionary. 27th Edition. 2000. Lippincott Williams & Wilkins, 351 West Camden Street, Baltimore, Maryland 21201.

Steen, Erik A. 1998. Complex Visual Hallucinations and Macular Degeneration. http://hubel.sfasu.edu/courseinfo/SL98/macdegen.html.

Stricker, R. B., and E. E. Winger. 2003. Musical Hallucinations in Patients with Lyme Disease. Department of Medicine, California Pacific Medical Center. South Med. J. 96(7):711-5.

Teunisse, Robert J., et. al. 1996. Visual Hallucinations in Psychologically Normal People: Charles Bonnet's Syndrome. The Lancet, Vol. 347. p. 794-97. http://www.geocities.com/franzbardon/CharlesBonnetSyndrome_e.html.

Thorpe, Lilian. 1997. The Treatment of Psychotic Disorders in Late Life. Can. J. Psychiatry 1997;42 Suppl. 1:19S-27S. http://www.cpa-apc.org/Publications/Archives/PDF/1997/June/supp/SUP1-04.PDF.

Tinnitus. ~2004. The Hearing Center. Fort Wayne, IN. http://www.hearingclinics.com/PDF_Files/Tinnitus.pdf.

Troost, B. Todd. ~2003. Central Auditory Disorders. http://ivertigo.net/hearing/hrcen.html.

Wade, Dr. Phillip S. 1995. Tinnitus Update–1995. In: *Vibes*. December, 1995. The Canadian Hearing Society, 271 Spadina Road, Toronto, Ontario M5R 2V3.

Zimmer, Carl. 2004. Can't Get it Out of My Head: Brain Disorder Causes Mysterious Music Hallucinations. The Sunday Telegraph Magazine. February 28. http://www.carlzimmer.com/articles/2004/articles_2004_Music.html.

Other **GuidePost** books in the series:

Everything You Wanted to Know About Your Hearing Loss But Were Afraid to Ask
(Because You Knew You Wouldn't Hear the Answers Anyway!)
by Neil G. Bauman, Ph.D.

If you have enjoyed this book and would like to learn more about hearing loss and how you can successfully live with it, you may be interested in some of the other helpful books in this series. Each book is packed with the things you need to know in order to thrive in spite of your various hearing loss issues.

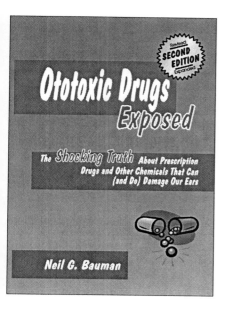

"Ototoxic Drugs Exposed—Prescription Drugs and Other Chemicals That Can (and Do) Damage Our Ears" ($39.99)

This book, now in its second edition, reveals the shocking truth that many prescription drugs can damage your ears. Some drugs slowly and insidiously rob you of your hearing, cause your ears to ring or destroy your balance. Other drugs can smash your ears in one fell swoop, leaving you with profound, permanent hearing loss and bringing traumatic change into your life. Learn how to protect your ears from the ravages of ototoxic drugs and chemicals. Describes the ototoxic effects of 743 drugs and 148 chemicals (634 pages).

When Hearing Loss Ambushes Your Ears—Here's What Happens When Your Hearing Goes on the Fritz ($10.75)

Hearing loss often blind-sides you. As a result, your first step should be to learn as much as you can about your hearing loss; then you will be able to cope better. This most interesting book explains how your ears work, the causes of hearing loss, what you can expect to hear with different levels of hearing loss and why you often can't understand what you hear. Lots of audiograms and charts help make things clear. You will also discover a lot of fascinating things about how loud noises damage your ears (56 pages).

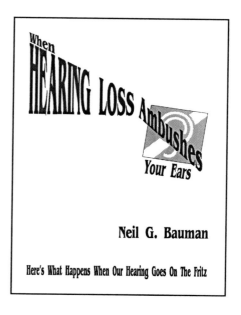

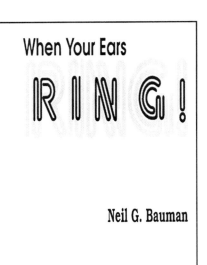

When Your Ears Ring! Cope with Your Tinnitus—Here's How ($10.75)

If your ears ring, buzz, chirp, hiss or roar, you know just how annoying tinnitus can be. You do not have to put up with this racket for the rest of your life. Recent studies show that a lot of what we thought we knew about tinnitus is not true at all. Exciting new research reveals what you can do to eliminate or greatly reduce the severity of your tinnitus. In this book you will learn what causes tinnitus in the first place and the steps you can take to bring it under control (56 pages).

Please Make My World Stop Spinning—The Agony of Meniere's Disease ($7.65)

Meniere's Disease is one of the more incapacitating things you can experience. If you suffer from your world spinning and have a fluctuating hearing loss together with noises in your ears, this book is for you. It explains what is known about Meniere's, its causes and the best treatments available today. There are lots of hints that you can try out for yourself to reduce or eliminate the effects of Meniere's disease. Since everyone is different, see what works for you (28 pages).

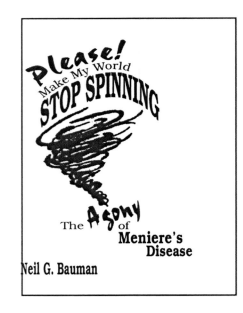

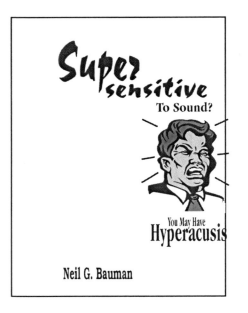

Supersensitive to Sound? You May Have Hyperacusis ($7.40)

If some (or all) normal sounds seem so loud they blow your socks off, this is the book you want to read! You don't have to avoid noise or lock yourself away in a soundproof room. Exciting new research on this previously baffling problem reveals what you can do to help bring your hyperacusis under control (24 pages).

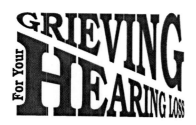

Grieving for Your Hearing Loss—The Rocky Road from Denial to Acceptance ($9.95)

When you lose your hearing you need to grieve. This is not optional—but critical to your continued mental and physical health. This book leads you through the process of dealing with the grief and pain you experience as a result of your hearing loss. It explains what you are going through each step of the way. It gives you hope when you are in the depths of despair and depression. It shows you how you can lead a happy vibrant life again in spite of your hearing loss. This book has helped many (40 pages).

Talking with Hard of Hearing People—Here's How to Do It Right! ($7.65)

Talking is important to all of us. When communciation breaks down, we all suffer. For hard of hearing people this happens all the time. This book is for you—whether you are hearing or hard of hearing! It explains how to communicate with hard of hearing people in one-to-one situations, in groups and meetings, in emergency situations, and in hospitals and nursing homes. When you use the principles given in this book, good things will happen and you will finally be able to have a comfortable chat with a hard of hearing person (28 pages).

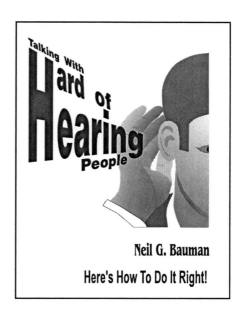

Hear! Here! You and Your Hearing Loss/You and Your Hearing Aids ($9.95)

Part I of this book contains a series of my newspaper acticles on hearing loss such as, "Hear Today. Gone Tomorrow?" "Hearing Loss Is Sneaky!" "The Wages of Din Is Deaf!" "When Your Ears Ring..." "Get In My Face Before You Speak!" "How's That Again?" "Being Hard of Hearing Is Hard" "I'm Deaf, Not Daft!" Part II contains articles on hearing aids such as, "You Better Watch Out..." "Before Buying Your First Hearing Aid..." "Please Don't Lock Me Away in Your Drawer" "Good-bye World of Silence!" "Becoming Friends with Your Hearing Aids" "Two's Better Than One!" (44 pages).

Coming Next: watch for this new book

Broken Ears—Wounded Hearts

Learn why hard of hearing people feel
and act the way they do. This book
discusses the emotional and psychological aspects of being hard of hearing
in a hearing world.

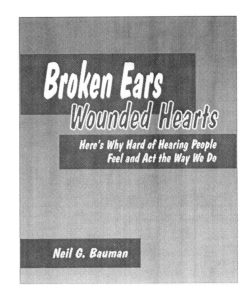

You can order any of these books (plus you can read other
helpful information about hearing loss) from the **Center for
Hearing Loss Help** web site at: http://www.hearinglosshelp.com
or place your order with GuidePost Publications (address below).

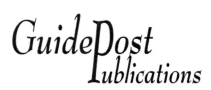

49 Piston Court,
Stewartstown, PA 17363-8322
Phone: (717) 993-8555
E-mail: info@GuidePostPublications.com
Website: http://www.GuidePostPublications.com

1134380